PEN

EXPEC

Emily Oster is a professor of economics at Brown University. She was a speaker at the 2007 TED conference and her work has been featured in *The New York Times*, *The Wall Street Journal*, *Forbes*, and *Esquire*. Oster is married to economist Jesse Shapiro and is also the daughter of two economists. She has two children, Penelope and Finn.

Praise for *Expecting Better*

"*Expecting Better* will be a revelation for curious mothers-to-be whose doctors fail to lay out the pros and cons of that morning latte, let alone discuss real science. And it makes for valuable homework before those harried ob-gyn appointments, even for lucky patients whose doctors are able to talk about the rationale behind their advice." —*The New York Times*

"Emily Oster combs through hundreds of medical studies to debunk many widely followed dictates: no alcohol, no caffeine, no changing the kitty litter. Her conclusions are startling. . . . *Expecting Better* walks women through medical literature surrounding every stage of pregnancy, giving them data to make informed decisions about their own pregnancy." —*New York Magazine*

"It seems that everyone—doctors, yoga teachers, mothers-in-law, and checkout ladies at grocery stores—are members of the pregnancy police. Everyone has an opinion. But not everyone is Emily Oster, a Harvard-trained economics professor at the University of Chicago. . . . To help the many women who reached out to Oster for advice, she compiled her conclusions in her new book, *Expecting Better*, which she describes as a kind of pregnancy 'by the numbers.'" —*New York Post*

"[Oster took] a deep dive into research covering everything from wine and weight gain to prenatal testing and epidurals. What she found was some of the mainstays of pregnancy advice are based on inconclusive or downright faulty science." —Associated Press

"Economist and author Emily Oster contradicts conventional wisdom and advocates a much more relaxed approach to pregnancy."
—*Daily Mail* (London)

"She's such a brilliant researcher and wordsmith." —Parents.com

"[*Expecting Better*] offers expectant mothers a new route to the delivery room."   —*The Times* (London)

"A comprehensive and lively debunking of the myths surrounding pregnancy."   —*The Telegraph* (UK)

"It took someone as smart as Emily Oster to make it all this simple. She cuts through the thicket of anxiety and received wisdom, and gives us the facts. *Expecting Better* is both enlightening and calming. It almost makes me want to get pregnant."
                —Pamela Druckerman, *New York Times* bestselling author of *Bringing Up Bébé* and *Bébé Day by Day*

"*Expecting Better* is a fascinating and reassuring tour of pregnancy and childbirth, with data leading the way at every juncture. From start to finish, Oster easily leads us through the key findings of the extant pregnancy-related research. My only regret is that my wife and I had three children without the benefit of this insightful approach."
                —Charles Wheelan, *New York Times* bestselling author of *Naked Statistics*

"The only antidote to pregnancy anxiety is facts, and Emily Oster has them in spades. Disarmingly personal and easy to read, this book is guaranteed to cut your freaking out in half. Pregnancy studies has a new heroine. Every pregnant woman will cheer this book—and want to take Oster out for a shot of espresso."
                —Rachel Simmons, *New York Times* bestselling author of *Curse of the Good Girl*

"This is a fascinating—and reassuring—look at the most important numbers of your pregnancy. It will make parents-to-be rethink much of the conventional wisdom: think bed rest is a good idea? Think again. This may be the most important book about pregnancy you read."
                —Steven D. Levitt, *New York Times* bestselling coauthor of *Freakonomics*

Expecting
Better

. . .

WHY THE CONVENTIONAL PREGNANCY
WISDOM IS WRONG—AND WHAT YOU
REALLY NEED TO KNOW

Emily Oster

PENGUIN BOOKS

PENGUIN BOOKS
An imprint of Penguin Random House LLC
375 Hudson Street
New York, New York 10014
penguin.com

First published in the United States of America by The Penguin Press,
a member of Penguin Group (USA) Inc., 2013
Published in Penguin Books 2014
This edition with revisions to chapter 8 published 2016

THE LIBRARY OF CONGRESS HAS CATALOGED
THE HARDCOVER EDITION AS FOLLOWS:

Oster, Emily.
Expecting better : why the conventional pregnancy wisdom is wrong—and
what you really need to know / Emily Oster.
pages   cm
Includes bibliographical references and index.
ISBN 978-1-59420-475-3(hc.)
ISBN 978-0-14-312570-9 (pbk.)
1. Pregnancy—Health aspects.   2. Pregnant women—Health and hygiene.
3. Prenatal care.   I. Title.
RG525.O87 2013
618.2—dc23
2012039780

Printed in the United States of America
9   10   8

Book design by Gretchen Achilles

To my sweet Penelope, who inspired this book,

and to my *mormor,*

who would have loved to meet her.

Acknowledgments

Thank you, first, to my wonderful book team. My agent, Suzanne Gluck, without whom this project definitely would not have gotten past chapter 1 and who tells me straight up when it's not quite there yet. Ginny Smith is some kind of secret genius editor who got this turned into a real book when I wasn't even looking. Thanks to her, Ann Godoff, and the whole team at Penguin for enormous support, genius title creation, and all sorts of other things.

Huge thank you to Jenna Robins, who read everything first, rewrote most of it, made me sound like less of an economist, and without whose help I never would have gotten off the ground.

Emily L. Seet, MD, was an incredible medical editor (although any mistakes remain very much my own). Emily Carmichael created lovely graphs with little guidance. Jen Taylor provided invaluable contracting assistance.

I am grateful to all my ladies, most of whom helpfully got pregnant at the same time and shared their stories (sometimes without knowing they'd be book fodder): Yael Aufgang, Jenny Farver, Hilary Friedman, Aude Gabory, Dwyer Gunn, Katie Kinzler,

Claire Marmion, Divya Mathur, and, most especially, Jane Risen, Heather Caruso, Elena Zinchenko, and Tricia Patrick.

Many colleagues and friends supported the idea and reality of this book at various stages. Including but by no means limited to: Judy Chevalier, John Friedman, Matt Gentzkow, Steve Levitt, Andras Ladanyi, Emir Kamenica, Matt Notowidigdo, Dave Nussbaum, Melina Stock, Andrei Shleifer, Nancy Zimmerman, and the More Dudes.

Actually putting the time into writing this would not have been possible without the help of many, many people in running my household. Most important of all, Mardele Castel, who has been Penelope's *Madu* since day one, who makes Penelope happy and her parents relaxed, and who, very simply, makes it all work.

I'm lucky to have an incredibly supportive family. Thank you to the Shapiros: Joyce, Arvin, and Emily. To the Fairs and Osters: Steve, Rebecca, John, and Andrea. And to my parents: I couldn't ask for better ones; Penelope is lucky to have you as her *mormor* and Grandpa Ray. Mom, I hope you feel the ninety-six hours of labor was worth it.

Finally, thank you to Jesse and Penelope, who, it goes without saying, were essential. You two make me happy every day. Penelope, you have the absolute best dad. I love you.

Contents

The Second Trimester

10. Eating for Two? You Wish 133
11. Pink and Blue 147
12. Working Out and Resting Up 152
13. Drug Safety 164

PART 4

The Third Trimester

14. Premature Birth (and the Dangers of Bed Rest) 179
15. High-Risk Pregnancy 187
16. I'm Going to Be Pregnant Forever, Right? 194
17. Labor Induction 201

PART 5

Labor and Delivery

18. The Labor Numbers 217
19. To Epidural or Not to Epidural? 225
20. Beyond Pain Relief 237
21. The Aftermath 255
22. Home Birth: Progressive or Regressive?
    And Who Cleans the Tub? 262
    Epilogue 274

Appendix: Quick Reference:
OTC and Prescription Drugs 277
Notes 282
Index 303

Introduction

In the fall of 2009 my husband, Jesse, and I decided to have a baby. We were both economics professors at the University of Chicago. We'd been together since my junior year of college, and married almost five years. Jesse was close to getting tenure, and my work was going pretty well. My thirtieth birthday was around the corner.

We'd always talked about having a family, and the discussion got steadily more serious. One morning in October we took a long run together and, finally, decided we were ready. Or, at the very least, we probably were not going to get any more ready. It took a bit of time, but about eighteen months later our daughter, Penelope, arrived.

I'd always worried that being pregnant would affect my work—people tell all kinds of stories about "pregnancy brain," and missing weeks (or months!) of work for morning sickness. As it happens, I was lucky and it didn't seem to make much difference (actually having the baby was another story).

But what I didn't expect at all is how much I would put the tools of my job as an economist to use during my pregnancy. This may seem odd. Despite the occasional use of "Dr." in front of my name, I am not, in fact, a real doctor, let alone an obstetrician. If you have a traditional view of economics, you're probably thinking of Ben Bernanke making Fed policy, or the guys creating financial derivatives at Goldman Sachs. You would not go to Alan Greenspan for pregnancy advice.

But here is the thing: the tools of economics turn out to be enormously useful in evaluating the quality of information in *any* situation. Economists' core decision-making principles are applicable everywhere. *Everywhere.* And that includes the womb.

When I got pregnant, I pretty quickly learned that there is a lot of information out there about pregnancy, and a lot of recommendations. But neither the information nor the recommendations were all good. The information was of varying quality, and the recommendations were often contradictory and occasionally infuriating. In the end, in an effort to get to the good information—to really figure out the truth—and to make the right decisions, I tackled the problem as I would any other, with economics.

At Chicago (and, now, Brown University) I taught introductory microeconomics. My students would probably tell you the point of the class is to torture them with calculus. In fact, I have a slightly more lofty goal. I want to teach them decision making. Ultimately, this is what microeconomics is: decision science—a way to structure your thinking so you make good choices.

I try to teach them that making good decisions—in business, and in life—requires two things. First, they need all the information about the decision—they need the right data. Second, they need to think about the right way to weigh the pluses and minuses of the decision (in class we call this *costs and benefits*) for them personally. The key is that even with the same data, this second part—this weighing of the pluses and minuses—may result in different decisions for different people. Individuals may value the same thing differently.

For my students, the applications they care about most are

business-related. They want to answer questions like, should I buy this company or not? I tell them to start with the numbers: How much money does this company make? How much do you expect it to make in the future? This is the data, the information part of the decision.

Once they know that, they can weigh the pluses and minuses. Here is where they sometimes get tripped up. The plus of buying is, of course, the profits that they'll make. The minus is that they have to give up the option to buy something else. Maybe a better company. In the end, the decision rests on evaluating these pluses and minuses *for them personally*. They have to figure out what else they could do with the money. Making this decision correctly requires thinking hard about the alternative, and that's not going to be the same for everyone.

Of course, most of us don't spend a lot of time purchasing companies. (To be fair, I'm not sure this is always what my students use my class for, either—I recently got an e-mail from a student saying that what he learned from my class was that he should stop drinking his beer if he wasn't enjoying it. This actually is a good application of the principle of sunk costs, if not the primary focus of class.) But the concept of good decision making goes far beyond business.

In fact, once you internalize economic decision making, it comes up everywhere.

When Jesse and I decided we should have a baby, I convinced him that we had to move out of our third-floor walk-up. Too many steps with a stroller, I declared. He agreed, as long as I was willing to do the house shopping.

I got around to it sometime in February, in Chicago, and I trekked in the snow to fifteen or sixteen seemingly identical houses. When I finally found one that I liked (slightly) more than the others, the fun started. We had to make a decision about how much to offer for it.

As I teach my students, we started with the data: we tried to figure out how much this particular house was worth in the market. This wasn't too difficult. The house had last sold in 2007, and we found the price listed online. All we had to do was figure out how much prices had changed in the last two years. We were right in the middle of a housing crisis—hard to miss, especially for an economist—so we knew prices had gone down. But by how much?

If we wanted to know about price changes in Chicago overall we could have used something called the Case-Shiller index, a common measure of housing prices. But this was for the whole city—not just for our neighborhood. Could we do better? I found an online housing resource (Zillow.com) that provided simple graphs showing the changes in housing prices by neighborhood in Chicago. All we had to do was take the old price, figure out the expected change, and come up with our new price.

This was the data side of the decision. But we weren't done. To make the right decision we still needed the pluses and minuses part. We needed to think about how much *we* liked this house relative to other houses. What we had figured out was the market price for the house—what we thought other people would want to pay, on average. But if we thought this house was really special, really perfect, and ideal for us in particular, we would probably want to bid *more* than we thought it was worth in the market— we'd be willing to pay something extra because our feelings about this house were so strong.

There wasn't any data to tell us about this second part of the decision; we just had to think about it. In the end, we thought that, for us, this house seemed pretty similar to all the other ones. We bid the price we thought was correct for the house, and we didn't get it. (Maybe it was the pricing memo we sent with our bid? Hard to say.) In the end, we bought another house we liked just as much.

But this was just our personal situation. A few months later one of our friends fell in love with one particular house. He thought this house was a one-of-a-kind option, perfect for him and his family. When it came down to it, he paid a bit more than the data might have suggested. It's easy to see why that's also the right decision, once you use the right decision process—the economist's decision process.

Ultimately, as I tell my students, this isn't just one way to make decisions. It is the *correct* way.

So, naturally, when I did get pregnant I thought this was how pregnancy decision making would work, too. Take something like amniocentesis. I thought my doctor would start by outlining a framework for making this decision—pluses and minuses. She'd tell me the plus of this test is you can get a lot of information about the baby; the minus is that there is a risk of miscarriage. She'd give me the data I needed. She'd tell me how much extra information I'd get, and she'd tell me the exact risk of miscarriage. She'd then sit back, Jesse and I would discuss it, and we'd come to a decision that worked for us.

This is not what it was like *at all*.

In reality, pregnancy medical care seemed to be one long list of rules. In fact, being pregnant was a lot like being a child again. There was always someone telling you what to do. It started right away. "You can have only two cups of coffee a day." I wondered why—what were the minuses (I knew the pluses—I love coffee!)? What did the numbers say about how risky this was? This wasn't discussed anywhere.

And then we got to prenatal testing. "The guidelines say you should have an amniocentesis only if you are over thirty-five." Why is that? Well, those are the rules. Surely that differs for different people? Nope, apparently not (at least according to my doctor).

Pregnancy seemed to be treated as a one-size-fits-all affair. The way I was used to making decisions—thinking about my personal preferences, combined with the data—was barely used at all. This was frustrating enough. Making it worse, the recommendations I read in books or heard from friends often contradicted what I heard from my doctor.

Pregnancy seemed to be a world of arbitrary rules. It was as if when we were shopping for houses, our realtor announced that people without kids do not like backyards, and therefore she would not be showing us any houses with backyards. Worse, it was as if when we told her that we actually *do* like backyards she said, "No, you don't, this is the rule." You'd fire your real estate agent on the spot if she did this. Yet this is how pregnancy often seemed to work.

This wasn't universal, of course; there were occasional decisions to which I was supposed to contribute. But even these seemed cursory. When it came time to think about the epidural, I decided not to have one. This wasn't an especially common choice, and the doctor told me something like, "Okay, well, you'll probably get one anyway." I had the appearance of decision-making authority, but apparently not the reality.

I don't think this is limited to pregnancy—other interactions with the medical system often seem to be the same way. The recognition that patient preferences might differ, which might play an important role in deciding on treatment, is at least sometimes ignored. At some point I found myself reading Jerome Groopman and Pamela Hartzband's book, *Your Medical Mind: How to Decide What Is Right for You,* and nodding along with many of their stories about people in other settings—prostate cancer, for example—who should have had a more active role in deciding which particular treatment was right for them.

But, like most healthy young women, pregnancy was my first sustained interaction with the medical system. It was getting pretty frustrating. Adding to the stress of the rules was the fear of what might go wrong if I did not follow them. Of course, I had no way of knowing how nervous I should be.

I wanted a doctor who was trained in decision making. In fact, this isn't really done much in medical schools. Appropriately, medical school tends to focus much more on the mechanics of being a doctor. You'll be glad for that, as I was, when someone actually has to get the baby out of you. But it doesn't leave much time for decision theory.

It became clear quickly that I'd have to come up with my own framework—to structure the decisions on my own. That didn't seem so hard, at least in principle. But when it came to actually doing it, I simply couldn't find an easy way to get the numbers— the data—to make these decisions.

I thought my questions were fairly simple. Consider alcohol. I figured out the way to think about the decision—there might be some decrease in child IQ from drinking in pregnancy (the minus), but I'd enjoy a glass of wine occasionally (the plus). The truth was that the plus here is small, and if there was any demonstrated impact of occasional drinking on IQ, I'd abstain. But I did need the number: would having an occasional glass of wine impact my child's IQ *at all*? If not, there was no reason not to have one.

Or in prenatal testing. The minus seemed to be the risk of miscarriage. The plus was information about the health of my baby. But what was the actual miscarriage risk? And how much information did these tests really provide relative to other, less risky, options?

The numbers were not forthcoming. I asked my doctor about drinking. She said that one or two drinks a week was "probably fine." "Probably fine" is not a number. The books were the same way. They didn't always say the same thing, or agree with my doctor, but they tended to provide vague reassurances ("prenatal testing is very safe") or blanket bans ("no amount of alcohol has been proven safe"). Again, not numbers.

I tried going a little closer to the source, reading the official recommendation from the American Congress of Obstetricians and Gynecologists. Interestingly, these recommendations were often different from what my doctor said—they seemed to be evolving faster with the current medical literature than actual practice was. But they still didn't provide numbers.

To get to the data, I had to get into the papers that the recommendations were based on. In some cases, this wasn't too hard. When it came time to think about whether or not to get an epidural, I was able to use data from *randomized trials*—the gold standard evidence in science—to figure out the risks and benefits.

In other cases, it was a lot more complicated. And several times—with alcohol and coffee, certainly, but also things like weight gain—I came to disagree somewhat with the official recommendations. This is where another part of my training as an economist came in: I knew enough to read the data correctly.

A few years ago, my husband wrote a paper on the impact of television on children's test scores. The American Academy of Pediatrics says there should be no television for children under two years of age. They base this recommendation on evidence provided by public health researchers (the same kinds of people who provide evidence about behavior during pregnancy). Those researchers have shown time and again that children who watch a lot of TV before the age of two tend to perform worse in school.

This research is constantly being written up in places like the *New York Times* Science section under headlines like SPONGEBOB THREAT TO CHILDREN, RESEARCHERS ARGUE. But Jesse was skeptical, and you should be, too. It is not so easy to isolate a simple cause-and-effect relationship in a case like this.

Imagine that I told you there are two families. In one family the one-year-old watches four hours of television per day, and in the other the one-year-old watches none. Now I want you to tell me whether you think these families are similar. You probably don't think so, and you'd be right.

On average, the kinds of parents who forbid television tend to have more education, be older, read more books, and on and on. So is it really the television that matters? Or is it all these other differences?

This is the difference between *correlation* and *causation*. Television and test scores are correlated, there is no question. This means that when you see a child who watches a lot of TV, on average you expect him to have lower test scores. But that is not causation.

The claim that *SpongeBob* makes your child dumber is a *causal* claim. If you do X, Y will happen. To prove that, you'd have to show that if you forced the children in the no-TV households to watch *SpongeBob* and changed nothing else about their lives, they would do worse in school. But that is awfully hard to conclude based on comparing kids who watch TV to those who do not.

In the end, Jesse (and his coauthor, Matt) designed a clever experiment.[1] They noted that when television was first getting popular in the 1940s and 1950s, it arrived in some parts of the country earlier than others. They identified children who lived in areas where TV was available before they were two, and compared them to children who were otherwise similar but lived in areas with no TV access until they were older than two. The families of these children were similar; the only difference was that one child had access to TV early in life and one did not. This is how you draw causal conclusions.

And they found that, in fact, television has no impact on children's test scores. Zero. Zilch. It's very precise, which is a statistical way of saying they are actually quite sure that it doesn't matter. All that research in public health about the dangers of *SpongeBob*? Wrong. It seems very likely that the reason *SpongeBob* gets a bad rap is that the kinds of parents who let their kids watch a lot of television are different. Correlation, yes. Causation, no.

Pregnancy, like *SpongeBob,* suffers from a lot of misinformation. One or two weak studies can rapidly become conventional wisdom. At some point I came across a well-cited study that indicated that light drinking in pregnancy—perhaps a drink a day—causes aggressive behavior in children. The study wasn't randomized; they just compared women who drank to women who did not. When I looked a little closer, I found that the woman who drank were also much, much more likely to *use cocaine.*

We *know* that cocaine is bad for your child—not to mention the fact that women who do cocaine often have other issues. So can we really conclude from this that light drinking is a problem? Isn't it more likely (or at least equally likely) that the cocaine is the problem?

Some studies were better than others. And often, when I located the "good" studies, the reliable ones, the ones without the cocaine users, I found them painting a pretty different picture from the official recommendations.

These recommendations increasingly seemed designed to drive pregnant women crazy, to make us worry about every tiny thing, to obsess about every mouthful of food, every pound we gained. Actually getting the numbers led me to a more relaxed place—a glass of wine every now and then, plenty of coffee, exercise if you want, or not. Economics may not be known as a great stress reliever, but in this case it really is.

More than even the actual recommendations, I found having numbers at all provided some reassurance. At some point I wondered about the risks of the baby arriving prematurely. I went to the data and got some idea of the chance of birth in each pregnancy week (and the fetal survival rate). There wasn't any decision to be made—nothing to really *do* about this—but just knowing the numbers let me relax a bit. These were the pregnancy numbers I thought I'd get from my doctor and from pregnancy books.

I've always been someone for whom knowing the data,

knowing the evidence, is exactly what I need to chill out. It makes me feel comfortable and confident that I'm making the right choices. Approaching pregnancy in this way worked for me. I wasn't sure it would work for other people.

And then my friends got pregnant. Pretty much all of them at the same time. They all had the same questions and frustrations I had. Can I take a sleeping pill? Can I have an Italian sub (I really want one! Does that make a difference?)? My doctor wants to schedule a labor induction—should I do it? What's the deal with cord-blood banking?

Sometimes they weren't even pregnant yet. I had lunch with a friend who wanted to know whether she should worry about waiting a year to try to get pregnant—how fast does fertility really fall with age?

Their doctors, like mine, had a recommendation. Sometimes there was an official rule. But they wanted to make the decision that was right for them. I found myself referring to my obstetrics textbook, and to the medical literature, long after my Penelope was born. There was a limit to the role I could play—no delivering babies, fortunately (for me and, especially, the babies). But I could provide people with information, give them a way to discuss concerns with their OBs on more equal footing, help them make decisions they were happy with.

And as I talked to more and more women it became clear that the information I could give them was useful precisely because it *didn't* come with a specific recommendation. The key to good decision making is taking the information, the data, and combining it with your own estimates of pluses and minuses.

In some cases, the existing rule is wrong. In others, it isn't a question of right or wrong but what is right for you and your pregnancy. I looked at the evidence on the epidural, combined it with my own plus and minus preferences, and decided not to have one. My friend Jane looked at the same evidence and decided to have one. In the end, I felt fine eating deli meats; my college room-mate Tricia looked at the evidence and decided she would avoid them. All of these are good decisions.

So this book is for my friends. It's the pregnancy numbers—the data to help them make their personalized pregnancy decisions and to help them understand their pregnancies in the clearest possible way, by the numbers. It's the suggestion that maybe it's okay to have a glass of wine and, more important, the data on why. It's the numbers on the risk of miscarriage by week, data on which fish to eat to make your kid smart (and which to avoid because they could make your kid dumb), information on weight gain, on prenatal testing versus prenatal screening, on bed rest and labor induction, on the epidural and the benefits (or not) of a birth plan. This book is a way to take control and to expect better.

I did the research for this book while pregnant with my daughter. A few years later, I found myself expecting again—a son this time. By this time the first edition of this book was out, and a number of people asked me whether this second pregnancy was any different. I told them, yes, it was a lot more relaxing since I didn't spend all my free time reading medical papers! But it turned out not to be entirely research-free. Between the two pregnancies the technology for prenatal screening changed a lot. I found myself revisiting my analysis there, and you'll hear more about my son, Finn, when you get to that chapter.

Pregnancy and childbirth (and child rearing) are among the most important and meaningful experiences most of us will ever have; probably *the* most important. Yet we are often not given the opportunity to think critically about the decisions we make. Instead, we are expected to follow a largely arbitrary script without question. It's time to take control: pick up a cup of coffee or, if you like, a glass of wine, and read on.

PART 1

In the Beginning: Conception

. . .

Prep Work

Some pregnancies are a surprise. If you're one of those women who woke up feeling queasy, took a pregnancy test on a whim, and were shocked to see the second pink line show up, congratulations! Please skip ahead.

But for a lot of us, we're thinking about getting pregnant long before it actually happens. I met my husband in college in 2001. We got married in 2006. Our daughter was born in 2011. I won't say I spent the whole ten years thinking about a baby, but I (and, later, we) did make a lot of choices with at least the long-term plan of having a family.

And as I approached 30, and pregnant friends started popping up here and there, I thought a little more seriously. I wondered if there was something I should be doing in advance, even before we started trying to get pregnant. Should I change my diet? My doctor did once suggest I should cut down on coffee, just so it wouldn't be such a shock to reduce when I was pregnant. Was that really necessary?

Mostly, I worried that I was getting old.

Thirty is not actually old in pregnancy terms. "Advanced

maternal age" is reserved for women over 35, and you wouldn't be faulted for thinking that 35 was a sharp cutoff. I read one paper once that referred to eggs as "best used by 35." Thanks, it's really helpful to know my sell-by date. But, of course, 35 is not a magical number. Biological processes don't work like this. Your eggs don't wake up on the morning of your 35th birthday and start planning their retirement party.

Starting pretty much the first day you menstruate, your fertility is declining. Your most fertile time is in your teens, and it goes down from there—30 is worse than 20, and 40 is worse than 30. But, of course, there are other factors that push you in other directions. I certainly wasn't in a good position to have a baby in my first year of graduate school at 23, and the truth is that I'd probably be in a better position at 35 than at 30.

It wasn't the only consideration, but I did wonder about how fast fertility declined. My doctor didn't seem worried—"You're not thirty-five yet!" she said—but that wasn't quite the detailed reassurance I was looking for.

I went looking for reassurance (or, at least, information) in the world of data, in the academic medical literature. As I expected, there was an answer. It just wasn't quite what the over-35 retired-eggs story would have suggested.

The main research on this uses data from the 1800s (it's old but the technology hasn't changed much!). Here is the idea: prior to the modern era, couples would pretty much get down to business right after the wedding, and there were limited birth control options. So you can figure out how fertility varies with age by looking at the chance of having children at all for women getting married at different ages.

Researchers found that the chance of having any children was very similar for women who got married at any age between 20 and 35. Then it began to decline: women who got married between

35 and 39 were about 90 percent as likely to have a child as those who got married younger than 35; women who got married between 40 and 44 were only about 62 percent as likely; and women who got married between 45 and 49 were only 14 percent as likely. Put differently, virtually everyone who got married between 20 and 35 had at least one child, compared to only about 14 percent of those who got married after 45.

You may or may not like to draw conclusions from such old data. People live longer now, and are healthier longer. It is certainly possible that as longevity and health increase, women will remain fertile longer. Even if you do take this data at face value, the reduction in fertility is not as dramatic as you might have feared. The 35- to 39-year-old group is only slightly less likely to have children; the major drop in fertility is not until after 40, and at least some women over 45 in this data did conceive—this in an era well before *in vitro fertilization* (IVF)!

Contemporary data looks fairly similar, perhaps even somewhat more encouraging. Researchers in France studied a group of around 2,000 women who were undergoing insemination with donor sperm. One nice aspect of this study is that they didn't have to worry that older people had sex less frequently because everyone in the study was trying to get knocked up at the right time of the month in a controlled environment. After 12 cycles, the pregnancy rate was around 75 percent for women under 30, 62 percent for women 31 to 35, and 54 percent for women over 35. In this oldest group things were similar for women 36 to 40 and over 40. More than half of the over-40 women in the sample got pregnant within a year.[1]

In the end, my doctor was basically right to pooh-pooh my worries. But for me, seeing the numbers this way, in black and white, was far more reassuring. I could see in detail that starting to try at 30 rather than at 28 was not going to make that much difference. I could think about the timing if we wanted, for example, more than one child. And I could see that the numbers were all pretty high—for me, reading "75 percent of women were pregnant with a year" was a lot more helpful than hearing things like, "It works out for most women." For one thing, how do I know if your "most" is the same as mine?

I'd experience this again and again. The value of having numbers—data—is that they aren't subject to someone else's interpretation. They are just the numbers. You can decide what they mean for you. In this case, it's true that it's harder to get pregnant when you are older. But it's not impossible, not even close.

When we did start thinking more seriously about a baby, I stopped focusing so much on age. (After all, what could I do? Not getting older is not exactly an option.) But I did wonder about other things I might do to prepare. I asked my OB at my yearly visit if there was anything I should be aware of. Other than some generic advice to relax (not one of my strengths), the one thing she focused on was exercise. Make sure you are exercising before you get pregnant.

When I talked to other women, it seemed like this was part of a more general theme—it's a good idea to try to be in good physical shape before getting pregnant. Independent of any medical advice, I had long harbored the fantasy of getting to my "goal weight" prior to pregnancy. I had achieved this weight exactly once in my life, before my wedding, through a process of five A.M. ninety-minute cardio workouts four days a week. I figured if I got to this weight again before we got pregnant, I'd be one of those Heidi Klum–type women who look great through the whole pregnancy and are back to bikini modeling eight weeks after giving birth.

In the end, of course, I got pregnant right after our summer vacation, not exactly the most weight-loss-friendly time of year.

That's okay, I figured, *I'm sure it will be easy to get to that goal weight after the baby is born.* I am nothing if not optimistic.

Other than some feeling of personal achievement, it wasn't clear to me why I should care about my prepregnancy weight. Does it matter for anything? A few pounds here and there, obviously not. Overall, yes. Women (and their doctors) worry a lot about weight gain during pregnancy, but it turns out that weight before pregnancy is much more important.

About 70 percent of the U.S. population are overweight (defined as a body mass index over 25), and 35 percent are obese (BMI over 30). (Note: to calculate your BMI, take your weight in kilograms and divide it by your height in meters squared. If you are 5 feet 6 inches and 150 pounds, your BMI is 24.2.) On a number of important dimensions, obese women in particular have more difficult pregnancies than normal-weight women.

One study that demonstrates this effectively used a group of roughly 5,000 births at one hospital in Mississippi.[2] The advantage of using a single hospital is that it means the women are all pretty similar in terms of income, education, and other characteristics. A large percentage of the women in the study were obese.

The authors looked at a very large number of outcomes related to the mothers: preeclampsia, urinary tract infection, gestational diabetes, preterm delivery, the need for labor induction, Cesarean delivery, and postpartum hemorrhage (bleeding after birth). They also looked at some things about the babies: shoulder dystocia (when the second shoulder gets stuck during delivery), whether the baby needed help breathing, the five-minute APGAR score (a measure of the baby's condition five minutes after birth), and whether the baby was abnormally small or abnormally large.

Obese women have more pregnancy complications, as the graph on the next page illustrates. One example: 23 percent of normal-weight women have a C-section, versus almost 40 percent

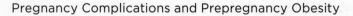

Pregnancy Complications and Prepregnancy Obesity

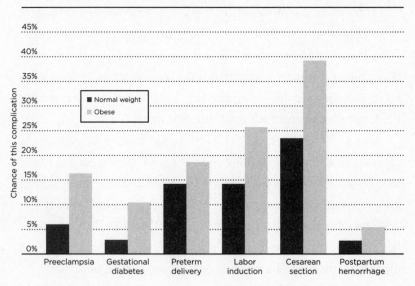

of obese women. The risk of preeclampsia, a serious pregnancy complication, is more than three times as high if you are obese. Overweight women (not in this graph) fall somewhere in the middle—a slightly higher risk for some complications, but the differences with normal-weight women are small.

When this study looked at infants, the babies of obese women were also more likely to have complications. If you are obese when you get pregnant, your baby is more likely to have shoulder dystocia, more likely to have low APGAR scores, and more likely to be abnormally large for gestational age. Even scarier, children of obese women are at higher risk for death, although this is *very* rare, regardless of Mom's weight.

This data is from just one study, but the findings are very consistent with other studies, from the United States and elsewhere.[3, 4] And the effects aren't limited to outcomes during pregnancy. Obese women have a harder time conceiving, and are more likely

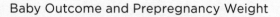

Baby Outcome and Prepregnancy Weight

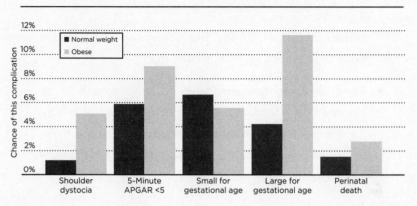

to miscarry early in pregnancy.[5] There is even some recent evidence that maternal obesity is associated with delays in breast milk coming in, which can impact breast-feeding success.[6]

A review article from 2010 summarizes the literature on this issue with a simple statement: "Maternal obesity affects conception, duration and outcome of pregnancy. Offspring are at increased risk of both immediate and long term implications for health."[7] In other words, it is harder to get pregnant, harder to sustain a pregnancy, more likely that later-term complications will arise, and more likely that there will be complications with the baby. All of which you would like to avoid.

None of this is to suggest that it's a problem if you can't lose that last five pounds, of course. The outcomes here are a result of pretty large differences in weight. I may have been disappointed not to get down to my fighting weight, but it is unlikely that it mattered. And being *too* skinny can also interfere with conception. But it does suggest that there are real benefits to getting your weight under control before you get pregnant. Of course, weight loss may have health benefits for reasons other than pregnancy. See, your (hypothetical) baby is helping out already!

The Bottom Line

- Fertility declines with age, but not as fast as you might expect—35 is not a magic number cutoff.

- Being obese before pregnancy is associated with an increased risk of complications for both you and your baby. Don't worry too much about a few pounds here and there, but if you are significantly overweight, weight loss before pregnancy may have benefits.

Data-Driven Conception

spent most of my twenties trying *not* to get pregnant. I used at least three versions of the birth control pill and even, for a brief time, something called "The Patch." So I knew I was really good at not getting pregnant. Of course, I worried that perhaps I wouldn't be so good at getting pregnant.

I'd like to say that I approached the process of conception in a laissez-faire way. After all, I was only thirty, we had plenty of time, and there was no indication that we'd have trouble conceiving. I wish I could say I was like my sister-in-law, Rebecca, who was so relaxed about this with my nephew that she was two months along before she even realized she was pregnant.

But this doesn't really fit with my personality. I suspected even before we got down to business that I would be a neurotic mess. I was correct. I actually had a panic attack about this *before we even started trying*. It must be a record. When I went to my primary care doctor, she looked at me thoughtfully and suggested that perhaps knowing more about the process would help me relax (even if I couldn't actually control it).

I don't know why this hadn't occurred to me before, but she

was exactly right. On her recommendation, I picked up a copy of *Taking Charge of Your Fertility* and read it cover to cover.

The main thing I learned was that a lot has to go right to get pregnant. It's kind of amazing that the human race continues to exist at all.

You probably remember the basics of conception from health class: unprotected sex, sperm meets egg, and, all of a sudden, you're pregnant. High school health class tends to give the impression that pregnancy is really, really likely—part of the general scare-tactic attitude. But, in fact, the majority of the time it is *not* possible to get pregnant. The key issue is timing: you need sperm to be around at the exact moment that the egg is ready.

When is that? The average woman has a menstrual cycle of 28 days, counting from the beginning of one period to the beginning of the next. The first day of your period is considered day 1. The week of your period and the week after it are preparation for ovulation. About 14 days after your period starts the egg is released (this is ovulation) and begins to travel down toward the uterus.

The egg is available for fertilization during this journey, which lasts a couple of days. If the egg meets a sperm on its way to the uterus and the sperm gets lucky, fertilization occurs. If you happen to release two eggs and they both meet sperm, you get twins; twins can also happen if the fertilized egg divides right at the beginning. When the fertilized egg (or eggs) reaches the uterus, implantation occurs and pregnancy actually begins. The process from egg release to implantation lasts 6 to 12 days. For most successful pregnancies, implantation occurs 22 to 24 days after the first day of your last period.[1]

This whole second half of the cycle (after the egg is released) is called the *luteal phase*. It's either taken up with fertilization and implantation (if you get pregnant) or with the egg waiting around in the uterus to be flushed out during your period. If you do not get pregnant, day 28 will bring your period. If you do get pregnant, day 28 will roll around periodless, and you'll be off and running. Here's the basic timeline (this is for someone with a standard 28-day cycle; if your cycle is a few days longer or shorter you might ovulate a bit earlier or later than day 14):

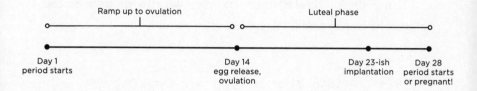

| Ramp up to ovulation | Luteal phase |

Day 1
period starts

Day 14
egg release,
ovulation

Day 23-ish
implantation

Day 28
period starts
or pregnant!

The key to pregnancy is that when the egg starts making its way down the tube, the sperm has to be waiting for it. This means the *best* time for sex or insemination is the day before or the day of ovulation. It takes some time for sperm to swim into the fallopian tubes, so the day after ovulation is generally too late.

Sperm are, however, a bit more robust than the egg. They can typically live up to 5 days in the fallopian tube, waiting. This means the window is actually a bit longer. Sex 4 or 5 days before ovulation can lead to a baby, although it's less likely. I was curious about how much less likely. All this talk about a small "ovulation window"—was there really any truth to that? How small was the window?

Figuring this out actually requires knowing quite a lot about people's sex lives. Fortunately, at least some researchers are up to the challenge. I found a study that followed more than 200 couples who were trying to conceive for more than a year. The authors recorded detailed information on when they had sex and collected their urine daily (daily!) so they could monitor both ovulation and pregnancy.[2] Using this information, the researchers figured out the best timing for baby-making sex (this wasn't the goal of the study, just an auxiliary fact we can learn from it).

What makes this question a bit tricky to answer is that most couples trying to get pregnant have sex frequently. This makes it hard to know which sex act led to the baby—was it the sex you had on the day of ovulation? Or three days before? The researchers get around this by focusing on women who had sex just one time in the plausible conception window.

Using these one-day-of-sex people, we can figure out the chance of conception by day. Here it is:

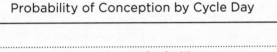

Probability of Conception by Cycle Day

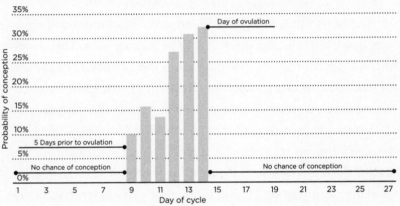

For most of the month, pregnancy is impossible (at least based on these data). No one conceived by having sex after ovulation—by the time the sperm gets up into the fallopian tubes, the egg is long gone. In addition, no one conceived by having sex more than 5 days before ovulation.

The window of possible conception is short: from 5 days before ovulation through the day of ovulation. But note that if you time it right, the chances of pregnancy are good. Conception rates are more than 30 percent for the day before and the day of ovulation! These odds are really not bad.

If you had to pick just one day in the month for sex, you'd want to pick the day you ovulate (or the day before: the pregnancy rates are similar). If you are using artificial insemination, it also makes sense to focus on the day before and the day of ovulation, when fertilization is most likely. For most women with a standard 28-day cycle, this is around the 14th day after your period starts.

Of course, one way to make sure that you definitely have sex on the day of ovulation is to have sex every day around the possible ovulation day (or just have sex every day). This technique is typically pretty popular with husbands, at least in the first month or two. But some OBs will warn you off this. I was told that the best strategy is to have sex every *other* day. If you did this, you'd be sure to capture at least one of the two best days, and the argument is that if you (or your partner) "save up" the sperm, then pregnancy chances are increased. On the other hand, saving them too much (say, skipping sex for more than ten days) tends to cause their effectiveness to diminish.[3]

This always sounded a little suspicious to me. I can easily believe that the amount of sperm is higher if you wait a day, but could it really be *more than twice as high,* which is what would have to be true for the every-other-day plan to beat out the every-day plan?

It turns out my skepticism was somewhat well placed. The same paper that gave me information on the right day for sex also determined whether frequency of intercourse mattered. The researchers calculated the predicted chance of pregnancy for people who had sex once during the 6-day window leading up to ovulation, for those who had it twice, three times, and so on. The chances were almost identical. In other words, there seems to be no benefit to alternating sex days, having sex more frequently, or having sex less frequently. The crucial thing is to hit the day of ovulation or the day before.

This appeared to make things simple. All I had to do was figure out when I was going to ovulate, and then have sex that day
or the day before. I figured this wouldn't be that hard, although I
worried a bit about work travel, and I patted myself on the back
for having avoided what the fertility book suggested was the
major infertility pitfall—namely, not having sex on the right day.

There was just one remaining problem: I didn't seem to be
ovulating at all. Or, at least, things didn't seem to be behaving
normally. When I went off the pill, my doctor said my cycle would
return to normal (or return to whatever it was before I went on
the pill, as if I could remember that). She said it would happen
within three months. It didn't. I went two months between periods, then had two within a few weeks.

I called the doctor at 3 months and 1 day. *What is going on?* I
asked the nurse when she called back. *Should I be worried? What
should I do?*

What I wanted was a concrete answer. Something like: 70 percent of women resume normal cycles within 3 months, 90 percent
within 6 months. I wanted to know whether it mattered that I had
been on the pill for 12 years. Would it take longer to get back to
normal? This is not what I got. What I got was best described as
vague reassurance (and the ever-helpful "Just relax!").

I thought if I pushed, I would get to the more detailed evidence,
but I didn't. "Everyone is different," I was told. "Yes, that is why
I asked about the *average*," I grumbled to Jesse. I would have this
type of experience again and again. How accurate is the prenatal
screening they suggested? "Quite accurate." When should I expect
to go into labor? "It's a different time for everyone."

I wanted a number. I craved evidence. Even if the answer was
that the evidence was flawed and incomplete, I wanted to know
about it. Yes, I understood that everyone was different. But that
doesn't mean there isn't any information!

Again, I headed out on my own to look for the numbers.

The most popular temporary forms of birth control in the United States are (in order): the pill, condoms, IUDs, and the withdrawal method. Obviously, neither condoms nor the withdrawal method have any impact on your menstrual cycle. If you've been using condoms, whatever cycle you've had up until now will continue. Same for withdrawal, and for any other barrier method (diaphragm, Today Sponge, etc.).

The pill makes things more complicated. As my doctor noted, sometimes the cycle returns to normal right away, but sometimes it takes a bit longer. The advantage of referring to the actual studies is that we can be more precise. In one study in Germany,[4] researchers studied menstrual cycles of women who just went off the pill. For some women it took up to 9 months to get back to a "normal" cycle. In the initial months after going off the pill these women had longer menstrual cycles, were more likely to have cycles in which they didn't ovulate, and were more likely to have cycles where the second half of the cycle (the luteal phase) was so short that pregnancy was unlikely.

This study is similar to others. Researchers in the United States studying women who had gone off the pill in the last 3 months found they had longer cycles (by a couple of days), more variable cycle length, and later ovulation in some cycles than those who had been off the pill longer.[5] In addition, when researchers measured their cervical mucus, the women who had been off the pill longer had cervical mucus that was more "welcoming" to the sperm.

The very good news, however, is that these effects are relatively short-lived. In the German study, virtually everyone had a normal cycle by 9 months after going off the pill. For some women it is much faster: 60 percent of women in that study had a normal cycle the first month off the pill.

I was also reassured that once you do ovulate, having been on the pill doesn't seem to impact pregnancy rates. In another

German study,[6] researchers studied women actually trying to get pregnant. They found that women who had just gone off the pill were slightly less likely to get pregnant in the first 3 months of trying, but no less likely to be pregnant within a year. This study also looked at the duration of pill usage and found no effect: even for people like me, who had been on the pill since their teenage years, things went back to normal in the same basic time frame.

What I took from this was that worrying at 3 months and 1 day was unnecessary. If I got to 9 months without things normalizing I could consider stressing out a bit.

Fewer women use IUDs, but the rates have crept up in the last decade. As with the pill, it takes a bit of time to recover fertility after using an IUD. In a recent literature review, authors found that women who had just gone off an IUD took (on average) a month longer to get pregnant than those who had just stopped oral contraceptives, but 80 to 90 percent (depending on the study) were pregnant within one year.[7]

So I waited, and a couple of months later things normalized a bit, just like the data said they would. But I still needed to figure out when I was ovulating. Day 14? Day 16? Day 12? Even after 6 months my cycle wasn't completely regular; I couldn't just assume it was day 14. Also, I quickly figured out that this was an opportunity to collect data. I couldn't resist!

There are three common ways to detect ovulation: temperature charting, checking cervical mucus, and pee sticks. The first two of these have been in use for many years; the pee stick method is relatively new.

Temperature Charting: Temperature charting (sometimes called BBT charting, for *basal body temperature*) relies on the mildly interesting fact that your body temperature is higher in the second half of the month, after ovulation, than before. You can therefore figure out when you ovulate by taking your temperature every day. The technique itself is not complicated. Every morning before you get out of bed (moving around affects your temperature; you ideally want to take it as soon as you wake up, before you do anything), you take your temperature using an accurate digital thermometer.

For the first half of the month, your temperature will be low—typically below 98 degrees. The day after ovulation, it will jump up, usually at least half a degree and sometimes more. This is the sign that you ovulated. Your temperature will stay high through the rest of the month, and then drop on the day your period starts, or (often) the day before. If you get pregnant, your temperature will stay high.

There are some very good things about temperature charting. In the month you are doing it, it can tell you with high certainty that you did, in fact, ovulate. If your cycles are regular, it can help you plan for the *next* month by showing you the day on which you generally ovulate. It can also tell you that you are pregnant. More than 14 days of high temperatures is a very good indication of pregnancy.

However, this isn't perfect. The biggest issue is that it tells you only *after* you ovulate. So although it is useful for predicting the next month, it doesn't help with this month. Also, it's not as simple as it seems. To really make this work you need to take your temperature at the same time every day, ideally first thing in the morning after four to five hours of continuous sleep. The results can get screwed up by jet lag, a fever, or a bad night of sleep.

I liked this method a lot, if only because it enabled me to feel like I was doing something proactive every day (and because it produced data, which I could use to make attractive charts). The downside is that I was never especially good at it.

My temperature chart from the month that I got pregnant with Penelope is on the next page. On one hand, the fact that my temperature eventually elevated and stayed up gave me a (small) clue that I was pregnant. On the other hand, all the jet lag and my

Basal Body Temperature Chart, June 2010

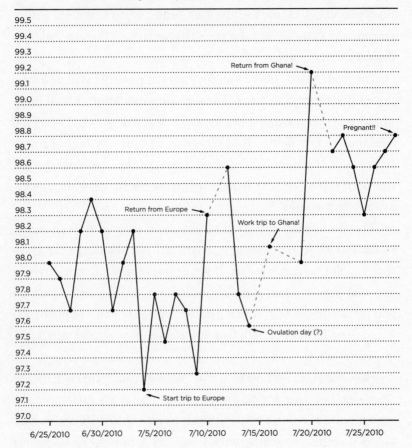

generally poor sleep meant that it was almost impossible to inter-pret. I initially thought I ovulated on June 9 because my tempera-ture went up on June 10; then I realized this was just because of the time change when we got back from Europe. The sustained higher temperatures did not occur until I got back from Ghana. The only way I knew that I must have ovulated before that trip was that Jesse wasn't there!

We can be a little more scientific about how useful this is for the average woman. In a study from the late 1990s,[8] researchers followed a set of women trying *not* to get pregnant and evaluated how good various methods were at detecting ovulation. In this study they were able to pinpoint the actual date of ovulation using ultrasound, so they knew the truth. The temperature-charting method as used by these women accurately identified the day of ovulation about 30 percent of the time. Another 30 percent of the time this method pointed to ovulation one day before it actually occurred.

That day before ovulation is also good for pregnancy sex. Putting this together: if you have sex on the date indicated by temperature charting, 60 percent of the time you would manage to time sex on one of the two most fertile days of the month.

Cervical Mucus: If you really want to get serious about natural ovulation detection, you probably want to chart your cervical mucus along with your temperature. This is a bit more complicated than temperature charting and, at least for some women (read: me), there is an "ick" factor. Here's the idea: right around ovulation your body produces a type of mucus ideal for sperm to swim through. You can detect this mucus in and around your cervix.

To do this, you reach into your vagina and run your finger around the cervix. This will collect some of the mucus, which you can test. Right before ovulation it will be stretchy, almost like egg whites. Days when you have this stretchy type of mucus are ideal for conception. The stretchiness peaks on the day of ovulation.

There are some pluses to this method. Unlike temperature charting, checking out your cervical mucus can tell you to try to conceive right now, versus telling you that you should have tried two days ago. It can be done any time of day, and works even if you sleep poorly, have a fever, etc. Many women use this in combination with temperature charting: assuming the two signs line up (i.e., you have the good type of mucus and a day or two later your temperature increases) you can get a very good picture of your cycle.

There are also minuses. The main one is that you may be uncomfortable mucking around in your vagina. A second issue is that semen can look a lot like high-quality mucus, so it's important to wait quite a while after sex (ideally a day or so) to do any checking. Even if you haven't had sex, it can be a bit hard to accurately classify the mucus "quality." For most women it takes a few months of practice to really figure it out.

Done correctly, cervical mucus is similar to body temperature charting in accuracy. In the same study that reported the accuracy of temperature charting, the researchers also had women identify their ovulation day based on cervical mucus. Actual ovulation day corresponded with the date identified based on cervical mucus in almost 50 percent of cases. In another study with a similar design,[9] but which focused only on cervical mucus, researchers found that monitoring mucus identified the day of ovulation in about 34 percent of cases and the day before ovulation in another 25 percent of cases.

Ovulation Detection Kits: Natural fertility charting has been around for decades. My mom remembers doing the temperature charting when trying to conceive my youngest brother (she claims she was no better at it than I was). It's cheap (a few dollars for a high-quality thermometer, maybe some graph paper), and can be quite accurate, especially once you get the hang of it.

But if you are after really accurate pinpointing of the day of ovulation, you probably want to go high tech: ovulation pee sticks. These work by detecting high levels of the *luteinizing hormone* (LH), which indicates ovulation. Using the pee sticks is simple. Starting around when you think ovulation is coming, you pee on a stick every morning. The stick will show you a line that darkens when the hormone levels are higher (some pee sticks use a digital readout instead). The hormone detected by this test is highest on the day before ovulation, so a positive result will tell you to try to conceive in the next forty-eight hours (that would be the day before and the day of ovulation) to maximize the chances of pregnancy.

The very significant upside of these tests is accuracy. In the same study that evaluated the temperature and mucus charting, urine-based ovulation tests put them to shame: these tests identified the day of ovulation 100 percent of the time. A study of the Clearblue fertility monitor specifically found that 23 percent of women who were randomly given access to this technology got pregnant in the two months of the study, versus only 15 percent who didn't have it.[10] Using these tests is also pretty easy: you pee on a stick, and that's about it.

The downside is cost. These tests run somewhere around thirty to forty dollars per month, multiplied by the number of months you need them.

There are a few even more high-tech options. For example, I briefly toyed with something called the OV-Watch. It looks like an ugly sports watch. You wear it for a few hours a day and it detects hormones from your skin. The idea is that it can detect even more hormones than the pee sticks, so it will tell you when you are approaching ovulation as well as when you ovulate. I could not get this to work. Apparently I sweat too much, or not enough, or at the wrong time.

Ultimately, virtually every woman I know has used at least some of these methods. Generally, people start with the temperature and move up to the pee sticks if a few months pass with no progress.

Are these helpful? The data suggest yes, but for me probably the biggest benefit was just that they gave me a way to feel in control. People say (correctly) that part of pregnancy and, especially, parenthood is giving up control. I just wasn't ready to do it quite yet.

The Bottom Line

- Timing matters! Pregnancy rates are high if you have sex on the day of ovulation or the day before, but fall rapidly away from that. It's possible to get pregnant by having sex as many as 5 days before you ovulate, but it's a lot less likely. After you ovulate, forget it until next month (you can still have sex, you know, for fun).

- It can take up to 9 months to resume your normal menstrual cycle after going off the pill, but there are no long-term effects on fertility.

- Low-tech ways of detecting ovulation (temperature charting, cervical mucus) are informative, but not 100 percent accurate.

- Higher-tech methods, such as ovulation pee sticks, are pricier but very accurate.

The Two-Week Wait

Here's the thing about trying to get pregnant. The first half of the month you spend carefully timing ovulation, taking your temperature, maybe peeing on a stick every morning. Then the second half of the month you . . . wait. You can't do anything to get pregnant once ovulation has come and gone. You can't yet figure out if you are pregnant. You're just in limbo.

And yet. You *might* be pregnant. Many women I know respected the "2-week wait" period: they acted as they would if pregnant for those 2 weeks. No caffeine, no drinking, no deli meats. This isn't such a loss if you're trying for only a few months, but at least one friend tried literally for *years* before using IVF to conceive her son, and she respected this 2-week wait period *the entire time*.

I succumbed to this pressure. I was careful about behavior in those 2 weeks. It was more than a little frustrating. My best friend and college roommate, Tricia, had a bachelorette party in Vegas during the second half of one month. I had two measly glasses of wine all weekend. A word to the wise: the "Thunder from Down

Under" is a lot less enjoyable without a bucket of Jell-O shots. Naturally, I got my period as soon as we returned.

After that weekend, I wondered if this was all really necessary. And what if you weren't trying to conceive, but it happened by accident, and you *had* joined in the Jell-O shots. How worried should you be?

The quick answer is that, assuming you did conceive, your behavior during those 2 weeks would have no impact on your baby (I can't believe I didn't figure this out before Vegas). The caveat is that it is possible that you could impact your chance of conception if you go *too* crazy.

The slightly longer answer relies on understanding how the baby develops at the very, very beginning. For the period between fertilization (around ovulation or a day or two later) and your missed period, your baby is a mass of identical cells. Any of these cells could develop into any part of the baby. If you do something that kills one of these cells (such as heavy drinking or some kind of really bad prescription drug use), another cell can replace it and do exactly the same thing. The resulting baby is unaffected. However, if you kill *too many* of these cells, the embryo will fail to develop and you will not wind up pregnant at all. It's an all-or-nothing thing.

Knowing this, I was slightly less careful in the post-bachelorette-party months. When I did turn up pregnant I certainly didn't worry about the night a week prior when I'd had 3 glasses of wine. Other friends didn't find this especially reassuring—in the service of taking every action to maximize the chance of conception, good behavior in the 2-week wait was just another thing. One friend admitted to compensating by getting drunk the day her period arrived each month. To each her own.

As the 2 weeks come to an end each month, there is the question of when to test. The pregnancy aisle at my local CVS boasts tests like First Response: Find out 5 days before your missed period! If you are counting, that's only about a week and a couple of days into the so-called 2-week wait.

It wasn't always like this. Historical pregnancy tests, like the modern ones, relied on urine. In ancient Egypt, women urinated onto various grains and evaluated their speed of growth. Faster growth equaled pregnancy. In the Middle Ages, the color of urine was evaluated to test for pregnancy. Oddly, these tests do have some limited predictive power, but probably not enough to be useful (for one thing, by the time the grain grows, you probably have figured out whether you're pregnant by other means!).

In the 1920s, doctors identified a hormone, hCG, that is secreted in the urine of pregnant women. A test was developed based on this, but it wasn't very user-friendly. It required injecting the urine into the ear of a live rabbit that was subsequently killed and dissected. It wasn't until the 1960s that doctors figured out how to test for this hormone without the rabbit.

The 1970s saw the introduction of the first home pregnancy tests. These required mixing your urine with other solutions in test tubes, leaving it for a few days, etc. These tests were not that accurate, and were too complicated and messy for most people. In those early days, women would typically realize they might be pregnant when their period was late, and then confirm with their doctor. This meant that by the time women actually got confirmation of pregnancy, they were about 5 weeks along. In the 1980s better home tests arrived (I dimly remember my mother using one with my youngest brother, born in 1985), but they still were not accurate until a week or 10 days after a missed period, so, again, pregnancy wasn't detected until about 5 weeks.

First Response puts this to shame, of course. The newer tests are able to detect pregnancy much earlier, by picking up a lower level of the hCG hormone than earlier tests did. As soon as the egg is fertilized, hCG is produced; the more sensitive the test, the sooner after implantation the test can show up positive.

It is worth noting that false negatives (that is, tests that say you are not pregnant but you actually are) are possible, especially if you are testing very early. Even the marketing materials for the most sensitive tests suggest that only about half of pregnancies are detected four days prior to a missed period. False positives, however, are very rare. If there are two lines, even if the second one is faint, you are pregnant. If the pregnancy is developing normally, the test line will probably get darker in the days after implantation as the hormone levels increase.

One downside to these more sensitive tests is that they are expensive. You can get a test that will work the day of your missed period for a dollar; the 5-day-in-advance tests cost more like ten dollars. I must have easily gone through one hundred dollars in these before one turned up positive.

The other thing to think about: you might not *want* to know. Pregnancy loss is very, very common at this early stage. As women find out they are pregnant earlier, the number who will subsequently learn that they have lost their pregnancy goes up. And it might go up by a lot. Some researchers suggest that as many as 50 percent or more of fertilized eggs do not result in pregnancy; of course, not all of these fertilizations are detected even with very sensitive tests.[1]

To get a sense of what number of pregnancies are lost very early, we can look at one study in the 1980s that followed women as they tried to get pregnant and tested their urine every day for signs of fertilization.[2] These researchers found that almost a quarter (22 percent) of pregnancies ended in miscarriage before pregnancy would have been detected using methods that were standard at the time. The researchers could detect these pregnancies using more sensitive tests. Given that miscarriage at this stage of pregnancy is similar to a heavy period, none of these women knew they were pregnant.

But the tests that the researchers were using in this case were similar in their sensitivity to what is now available in the most sensitive home pregnancy tests. This means that a lot of the pregnancies that ended in early miscarriage and would *not* have been detected in the 1980s now probably would be (or at least could be). If we take the numbers seriously, and everyone nowadays used the most sensitive home pregnancy tests, we could see miscarriage rates 22 percent higher than we did in the 1980s. But this is due to better detection, not because miscarriage rates have increased.

In addition, these early pregnancy losses, far from being harbingers of future fertility problems, actually are a good sign about fertility. In the same study, 95 percent of women who had a very early loss went on to have a recognized pregnancy. This was higher than for women who didn't have an early pregnancy loss.

Given this, it's worth thinking about whether those expensive early pregnancy tests are really worth it. You might be the kind of person who wants to know everything that is going on. But you also might rather wait and see.

The Bottom Line

- Very bad behavior during the 2-week wait could affect your chance of conception, but won't affect the baby if you do conceive.

- Early pregnancy tests can detect a pregnancy 4 or even 5 days before your missed period, but pregnancy loss is common in this period.

PART 2

The First Trimester

· · ·

4

. . .

The Vices: Caffeine,
Alcohol, and Tobacco

learned I was pregnant on day four of a weeklong summer economics conference. As usual, I couldn't tell whether my period was late or not—the temperature charting hadn't exactly cleared things up for me—but when I woke up at 6:45 feeling a little funny, I decided it was worth a shot. I had brought one First Response test to the conference, just in case. Amazingly, there were two lines.

I woke Jesse up immediately. He was happy, but groggy. He wondered why I hadn't let him sleep until his alarm went off at seven. Was there anything we needed to do right now? No? Then why get him up? He put a pillow over his head and fell back to sleep. (I took this to heart: four years later, when I learned I was pregnant with Finn, I notified him via a Google calendar invite to the due date.)

Obviously I wasn't going to go back to sleep. I opened my computer and started planning. I loaded up a little due-date calculator—April 1 or April 7, depending on whether I dated from last menstrual period or from the suspected conception day—and started browsing the Internet, looking for baby information. At some point I thought I'd go down to get a cup of coffee (Jesse had decided to sleep in after being so rudely awakened).

And then it hit me, of course. Could I even have coffee? Wasn't caffeine off-limits? I had spent a huge amount of mental energy up to this point thinking about getting pregnant and almost none on thinking about being pregnant (I didn't learn from this; it would come up again when I realized after Penelope was born that I hadn't done any research on what you do with the baby once it arrives).

This was urgent. The decision about coffee had to be made *now*. I could already feel a caffeine withdrawal headache coming on, and getting through an entire day of conference talks (especially day four) typically requires a pretty steady caffeine drip.

At the end of the day was the conference cocktail party and clam bake. I'd usually have a glass of wine while fighting with other economists over who gets seconds on lobster. Was that okay? The wine was not as urgent as caffeine, to be sure, but I did want to know. I'm not a smoker, but for women who do smoke, tobacco probably falls even higher on the "needs" list than coffee.

Finding information on the Internet about caffeine, alcohol, and tobacco during pregnancy is easy. There are official recommendations from national organizations, there are recommendations from specific doctors and books, and there are other people, on chat boards and blogs. There is no shortage of opinions, but there is a definite shortage of agreements.

Chat board debates about this devolve pretty quickly, and almost never involve any actual evidence. "I had a glass of wine every day and my baby is perfectly fine." "A friend of a friend did one champagne toast during pregnancy and has a developmentally delayed child." "My mother's coworker's sister's neighbor's daughter drank a six-pack a day and her son is a genius." "In France doctors prescribe wine to pregnant women." And on and on and on.

The fact that people on chat boards argue is a given (what else are these boards for?). What I found more surprising was that official recommendations disagreed with one another. In the case of alcohol, although all the pregnancy organizations in the United States recommend a policy of abstinence, similar organizations in some other countries indicate that occasional drinking is fine.

Caffeine is similar—recommendations differ across countries, yes, but also across books and across OBs within the United States. My OB said having less than 200 milligrams a day (about 16 ounces of coffee) was fine. My sister-in-law's OB told her no more than 300 milligrams. My best friend's said no caffeine. When we turn to books, the aptly named *The Panic-Free Pregnancy* takes the stance that caffeine in moderation (up to 300 milligrams) is fine. The *Mayo Clinic Guide to a Healthy Pregnancy* rules out caffeine in any dose, although notes that some OBs will say it is okay in moderation. It suggests switching to decaf. *What to Expect When You're Expecting* goes with the 200-milligram rule but indicates that you should check with your OB in case her recommendation differs. They also suggest that you check with your barista, because caffeine amounts differ by coffee provider!

Even if there had been a very consistent standard recommendation (as there is in the case of smoking), I still would have wanted to know what evidence backed it up. But my desire for evidence was made even more extreme by the fact that people disagreed. Was it 200 milligrams of caffeine, or 300 milligrams, or none? All these recommendations must have, in principle, been based on some data. It can't possibly have been the same data, though, or at least not the same interpretation.

It didn't take me long to realize that reading online advice about this—even official American Congress of Obstetricians and Gynecologists policy briefs—wasn't going to be enough to figure out the truth. I had to go to the source of the recommendations, to the academic medical literature. When I got into that, I saw why these recommendations differed so much and were so confusing: the quality of the medical research on this varies enormously.

And I quickly realized that a lot of the quality differences boiled down to exactly the issues I faced in my own research.

Economics is a pretty broad field (it would have to be to include both me and the guys who make policy at the Federal Reserve). In my particular subfield, most of the important questions involve trying to understand how changing one thing affects another. Among the last things I finished before getting pregnant was a paper about television and gender in India. The paper asked: if you give people in rural India access to cable television, does that change their attitudes toward women?

The goal of that study was to draw causal conclusions. At the end of the day we wanted to be able to say something like: "If we gave more people televisions, attitudes toward women would improve." One great way to do this would be to randomly pick some people to get televisions. You could watch them over time and see if their attitudes changed more than the people to whom you didn't give TVs. This method is called a *randomized trial*.

The name "randomized trial" is actually pretty descriptive. In a study like this researchers begin with a sample of people and randomly assign some of them to one treatment and some to another. If they were testing the efficacy of a new drug, for example, they would take a bunch of sick people and randomly give half of them the new drug and half nothing (or maybe a sugar pill). The key is that because the assignment is done *randomly*, the people who get the drug are similar to those who do not on every dimension *other than* using the drug. If they get better faster, you can conclude that the drug worked.

Randomized trials are used sometimes in economics, and much more in medicine. They are a tried-and-true method, and done correctly, you can be confident in drawing causal conclusions.

In fact, in some areas of pregnancy I was able to use data from trials like these. It made my decision making a lot easier.

But randomized trials are not always possible. In the case of our television study, it just wasn't feasible to assign televisions randomly. In the case of something like caffeine in pregnancy, the issues are ethical. Imagine an experiment in which some women are told to drink 9 cups of coffee a day and some are told to drink none. No ethical review board would approve that study (nor should they), and it's hard to imagine the pregnant woman who would want to participate (and not only because that's a gross amount of coffee!).

When researchers can't randomize, we are left trying to figure out these relationships using what is called *observational data*: comparing, say, pregnant women who drink coffee with those who do not. Or comparing families with televisions to families without them. It shouldn't be too hard to see where this might run into problems.

The TV example is easy to see. What kinds of people in rural India have televisions? The answer is rich people and those with a lot of education. It is definitely true that people with televisions have more liberal attitudes toward women than people without them. But is this because of television? Or because of education? It's well known that the more educated people in India tend to have more favorable attitudes toward gender equality. Could we really change attitudes toward women in rural India by giving people televisions, or would their attitudes be changed only by giving them more education (useful, but much harder policy)?

The same problem crops up in pregnancy research. Women who drink coffee during pregnancy tend to be older than those who do not. Say I told you miscarriage is more likely among women who drink coffee. Is that because of the coffee? Or is it because they are older? Could we decrease the miscarriage rate by taking away the coffee, or would you have to make people magically younger?

Getting around this problem successfully requires careful thought, careful study design, and good data. In the work on television, we avoided this by comparing the attitudes of the same people before and after they had access to television. Since we could see the same person "with television" and "without television," that helped us eliminate a lot of these problems.

You could imagine doing the same thing in pregnancy—look at the same women who drink coffee with one pregnancy and not with another—but I don't know of any data like this. Instead, in most of the studies of this question, the best they can do is use statistical analysis to adjust for basic differences across people— age and education, for example.

I quickly realized that some of these studies are much, much better than others.

This is where my training came in. There are literally hundreds of studies published in the medical literature on caffeine and miscarriage (this is the big concern with coffee during pregnancy). And from the outside, from the basic description, they all look pretty similar—comparing women who drank coffee with those who did not.

But when you get into the details, into the nuts and bolts, some of the papers are pretty good and some are terrible. Much of the time I invested in figuring all this out was spent trying to separate the wheat from the chaff: what studies can we learn something from, and which should we dismiss as totally uninformative?

And, oddly, I realized that training as a health economist was in many ways *better* than training in public health or medicine for this. Economists almost never have access to randomized trials. So we have developed techniques, statistical methods, to try to learn as much as possible from *non*randomized data. In graduate school I spent much of my time reading papers very much like this, trying to figure out which were good and which were not so good.

It took me longer than that first morning to wade through the papers. I pretty quickly realized that the official recommendations were extremely cautious, so I decided that sticking to them was safe until I figured it all out. I kept myself at 2 cups of coffee a day, and I avoided alcohol. This was added incentive to do the research fast.

Ultimately, I concluded that these recommendations were not just very cautious, they were *too* cautious. In moderation, pregnant women should feel comfortable with both alcohol and caffeine.

For alcohol, this means up to 1 drink a day in the second and third trimesters, and a couple of drinks a week in the first. In fact, for the most part studies fail to show negative effects on babies even at levels higher than this. By a drink here I mean a standard drink—4 ounces of wine, 1 ounce of hard liquor, 12 ounces of beer. No yard-long margaritas!

Caffeine is actually a little more complicated. I ultimately concluded that 3 to 4 8-ounce cups of coffee per day (more than many people drink, although actually not more than I drink) are fine. You might end up deciding you are comfortable with less, or with more; I'll try to make it clear in this chapter what the trade-offs are. There is no question that some coffee is no problem.

All the evidence I used for this is publicly available—accessible to anyone. That includes the people who make the official recommendations. So why did my conclusions differ from theirs? At least two reasons. One is overinterpretation of flawed studies. But the bigger thing, I think, is the concern (which was expressed to me over and over again by doctors) that if you tell people they can have a glass of wine, they'll have 3 (or one giant "bowl-o-wine"). Even if one isn't a problem, three are. Better to say you can't have any, as that rule is easy to understand.

I can see the argument here. But, to put it mildly, I'm not crazy about the implication that pregnant women are incapable of deciding for themselves—that you have to manipulate our beliefs so we do the right thing. That feels, again, like pregnant women are not given any more credit than children would be in making important decisions.

You may decide that you want to follow the national recommendations; that's fine. Or you may decide you share my conclusions that a drink and a shot of espresso are not a problem. This book is very specifically not about making recommendations; it's about acknowledging that if you have the right information you can make the right decision for yourself.

Although I will immediately contradict myself and make one recommendation (and back it up with evidence): do not smoke. This is the official line, and the data are squarely behind it. Smoking puts both you and your baby at risk.

Alcohol

When I was about 3 months pregnant and just starting to tell people about the pregnancy, I was hosting a party. A guest arrived and I offered to get him a glass of wine. He said, only half-joking, "You shouldn't even be carrying wine!" If you drink alcohol while pregnant (in the United States in particular) people feel free to judge you.

The restrictions and judgment are, very broadly, rooted in truth. Fetal alcohol spectrum disorders (FASD) refers to a range of mental and physical disabilities that can result from drinking during pregnancy. Physical symptoms include low birth weight, small head circumference, and facial abnormalities (flattened cheekbones and small eye openings). Cognitive symptoms come in a broader range: developmental delays, poor socialization skills, and learning difficulties.

There is no question that very heavy drinking during pregnancy is bad for your baby. Women who report binge drinking during pregnancy (that's more than 5 drinks at a time) are more likely to have children with serious cognitive deficits. In one Australian study, women who binged in the second or third trimester were 15 to 20 percentage points more likely to have children with language delays than women who didn't drink.[1] This is repeated over and over again in other studies.[2] Binge or heavy drinking in the first trimester can cause physical deformities, and in the later trimesters, cognitive problems. These problems can occur even with infrequent binges. If you are binge drinking, stop.

However, this does not directly imply that light or occasional drinking is a problem. When I looked at the data, I found no credible evidence that low levels of drinking (a glass of wine or so a day) have any impact on your baby's cognitive development.

This is probably surprising given the rhetoric around even occasional drinking during pregnancy in the United States, but it really shouldn't be. Think about Europe. Much of the continent is much more permissive about light drinking during pregnancy. Heavy drinking is frowned upon everywhere, but some places in Europe have recommendations suggesting that a few drinks a week are fine. An occasional glass of wine or beer is much more common there. Yet there is no evidence of more fetal alcohol syndrome in Europe; if anything, rates are higher in the United States.[*, 3] If having a couple of glasses of wine a week lowered IQ, we would see big differences between the United States and Europe. This is simply not the case.

This seems to reflect a lot of the differences in the attitudes toward drinking between the United States and elsewhere. When I go to conferences or talks in Europe it's common to have a glass of wine with lunch. Not to get drunk, of course. Just because it goes well with food. Perhaps because there it's more common to enjoy a drink in moderation socially, with a meal, people are more comfortable with the idea that you can, in fact, have one small

---

* It's hard to know why this is. As fetal alcohol syndrome is typically a result of binge drinking, it is possible that it could be due to the United States having more inequality in drinking—a lot of people not drinking at all and a few engaging in binge drinking— as opposed to other countries where most people drink moderately.

glass of wine and stop. This issue that doctors constantly mentioned to me—that women wouldn't be able to stop at just one—just comes up less.

And, in fact, although it's not so out in the open, I think occasional drinking is more common during pregnancy in the United States than we are led to believe. At the start of my second trimester, my doctor told me a couple of glasses of wine a week were fine. Most of my friends had a similar conversation with their doctors—"Don't overdo it, but if you want to have a glass of wine with dinner occasionally, that's fine." In surveys in the United States, about 40 percent of doctors do not always suggest complete abstinence during pregnancy.[4]

It's like a secret code. The problem, of course, with one official recommendation and a different "secret" recommendation is that no one really goes through the evidence for the latter. So you're left wondering: is this just your opinion that it's okay to have a drink, or is there some reason to think that it's actually okay?

To understand why there is a difference between excessive drinking and moderate or light drinking, it's useful to think a little bit about how the biology works. Many women seem to think that when they drink, that glass of wine is channeled directly to the fetus. People correctly note that you would not give your infant a glass of wine, so why would you give your fetus one? Needless to say, this is not really how it works.

When you drink, alcohol enters your digestive system and is passed into your bloodstream. Your liver processes the alcohol into a chemical called acetaldehyde and then into acetate. The acetaldehyde is toxic to other cells, and depending on how quickly you drink, it can remain in your bloodstream. You share your blood with your baby through the placenta; acetaldehyde, which remains in your bloodstream, is therefore shared with the fetus. Your baby actually can process some alcohol, but not as much as an adult (obviously). If too much acetaldehyde is passed to the baby, it can get into his tissues and impact development. When you drink slowly, you metabolize much of the alcohol before it would get to the fetus. If you drink quickly, your liver cannot keep up and toxins are passed to the fetus. This is why binge drinking is so bad, but it also illustrates why negative effects of light drinking do not follow directly from negative effects of heavy drinking.

If we want to learn about the impact of light drinking on pregnancy, we actually want to look at women who are light drinkers. We cannot look at studies of binge drinking and say, well, if 5 drinks at a time decreases your child's IQ by 10 points, then 1 drink will decrease it by 2 points. It simply doesn't work like that.

Once I realized this, I started scouring the medical literature for studies that looked specifically for impacts of light drinking. I mainly focused on studies that included women having up to a drink a day. I never felt the urge to have a whole bottle of wine at a sitting (I don't really feel this urge while *not* pregnant), or even to order a second cocktail. What I really wondered was: at the end of a long day, a few times a week, could I have a glass of wine?

For the most part, the studies I found all had a similar structure. There are no randomized trials here; the ethics are just too complicated. This means the studies compared women who chose to drink different amounts of alcohol. All these studies have the problem that the kinds of women who drink are different from those who do not. The key was to find the studies that had this problem the least.

One big worry about drinking during pregnancy is child behavior problems later. Among the best studies of the behavior issue is one published in 2010 in the *British Journal of Obstetrics and Gynecology*.[5] There are a few things that make this a reliable study: it's pretty large (3,000 women), and they collected information about maternal drinking *during* pregnancy (at 18 and 34 weeks). Asking people about their behavior while they are doing it tends to be more reliable than asking them to remember later on. The study also followed the children of these women from birth through the age of 14; they looked at behavior problems starting at age 2.

The other thing I liked about this study was that it was run in Australia, where recommendations on drinking during pregnancy are more lax than in the United States. Because drinking during pregnancy in the United States is judged so harshly, we worry when relying on data from the United States that only women who are reckless in other ways continue to drink. In Australia (and European countries), where people are more permissive, it's less likely that the variation in drinking reflects variation in other behaviors.

Women in the study were classified in five groups: no alcohol, occasional drinking (up to 1 drink per week), light drinking (2 to 6 drinks per week), moderate drinking (7 to 10 drinks per week) and heavy drinking (11 or more drinks per week). I ignored the last guys, as they were way above my cutoff of 1 drink per day.

Here's a visual of their results: the percent of children with behavioral problems by drinking amount. This graph shows the data for 2-year-olds in relation to drinking amounts at 18 weeks of pregnancy. The paper also illustrates behavior problems later on, and drinking at 34 weeks. It doesn't matter much: all the results look pretty much just like this.

Based on this picture and the more complex statistical analysis in the paper, there is no evidence that more drinking leads to higher levels of behavior problems. In fact, the statistics in the paper show that light drinkers (that's 2 to 6 drinks per week) are actually *significantly less likely* to have children with behavior problems than women who do not drink at all.

The other big concern with alcohol is low IQ. Again, my favorite study on this issue comes out of Australia. It has a lot of the same high-quality features: large study, drinking information

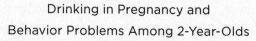

Drinking in Pregnancy and
Behavior Problems Among 2-Year-Olds

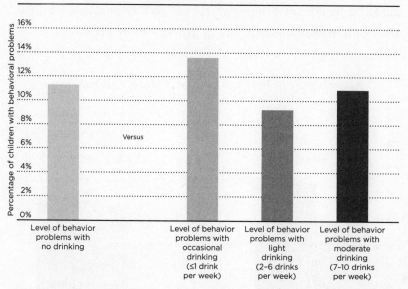

collected during pregnancy, long-term follow-up. And, of course, the fact that it was run in Australia. This study started in the early 1980s by asking about 7,200 pregnant women about their drinking during pregnancy. Roughly 5,000 of their children completed an achievement test at age 14.[6]

Drinking information was collected after the first 3 months of pregnancy and after the last 3 months. These authors define their drinking categories by the day: no drinking, less than ½ glass per day, ½ to 1 glass per day, and greater than 1 glass per day.

They measured IQ with a test called Raven's matrix. It works like most IQ tests in that higher scores are better, and the test is designed so that the average person will score 100. Here's the data:*

Just as in the study of behavior, there is no evidence here to suggest that the children of light drinkers are worse off than those

---

* This graph reports coefficients adjusted for maternal demographics and weight.

of women who drink nothing. In fact, their scores are higher on average (although these results are not statistically significant—they may just reflect random variation). The researchers concluded there is no evidence of worse test performance, even among the children of moms who have a drink or more per day.

Raven's Matrix Performance and Maternal Drinking

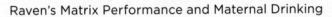

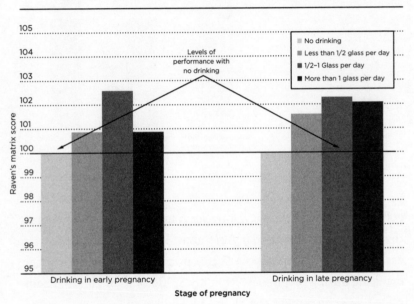

It's not just Australia (worth saying, lest you are tempted to conclude that Foster's is just very good for babies). A very similar study in England interviewed women in early pregnancy about drinking patterns and then gave their children an IQ test at age 8.[7] Same result: no impact of drinking on IQ.*

Perhaps somewhat puzzling, many of these studies actually

---

* This particular study observed a lot of information about children—including information on the drinking behavior of the father—and after adjusting for everything about the child, they still found that test scores were unaffected by maternal drinking in pregnancy.

find that women who drink moderately in pregnancy have children with higher IQ scores. Most researchers agree this effect is probably not causal, and may be due to the fact that women who drink moderately, at least outside of the United States, tend to be better educated than those who do not. Knowing this, you might be concerned that a negative impact of light drinking is being masked by the higher education.

The English study I mentioned above is a good antidote to this concern: the authors are able to use the drinking behavior of fathers to adjust for these baseline differences. And, reassuringly, they find no effect of light drinking on IQ. I pushed and pushed to learn the truth from this literature, and in the end I was surprised at how consistent the findings were. It's simply very, very difficult to find good evidence that a small amount of alcohol has any negative impact whatsoever on long-term child behavior or IQ.

When I was finishing edits on this chapter, my friend Hilary e-mailed me a link to yet another study. "Did you see this?!" was the subject line. It was a large study, run in Denmark, showing no impact of drinking up to 8 drinks a week on child IQ at age 5.[8] Articles written in the popular press acted like this was a huge surprise. I just threw it on the increasingly large pile of papers showing the exact same thing.

This is not to say that one cannot unearth studies that find that light drinking is a problem; the issue is that these studies are very deeply flawed. One that gets cited frequently was published in the journal *Pediatrics* in 2001.[9] On the face, this study looks similar to the ones I discussed above. Women were interviewed about their drinking during pregnancy, and were recontacted for a child-behavior assessment when the child was about 6. The study is a bit smaller (only about 500 kids), but otherwise you might think it was just as reliable as the ones I talked about earlier.

This study did find at least some evidence that lighter drinking impacts behavior. When the authors compared women who didn't drink during pregnancy to those who had one drink or less per day, they found more evidence of aggressive behavior (although not of other behavior problems) among the children of women who drank. The researchers concluded that even one drink a day causes behavior problems.

So what's the problem?

One of the very nice things about the previous studies—the ones I liked—was that the groups of women who drank different amounts were not *that* different in other ways. If this were not the case, we would be worried that the other differences among the women—not the drinking—were responsible for the behavior problems. This is not just some idle, esoteric, statistical concern. This is *the* concern about drawing causal conclusions.

This last paper failed on this count. In this study, cocaine use during pregnancy was reported by 18 percent of the women who didn't drink at all and 45 percent of the women who had one drink per day. Presumably your first thought is, really? Cocaine? Your second thought should be to note that the drinkers were also a lot more likely to be cocaine users.

This should give you pause. You should start to wonder: maybe the problem is that *cocaine* makes a child more likely to have behavior problems, not light drinking. Also, children of light drinkers were less likely to live with two parents than children of nondrinkers. Hmm. Maybe it's living with dad that matters for behavior (a fact that has been shown in many other contexts).

At this point, I threw that paper in the trash. Maybe if I was wondering about combining my end-of-day glass of wine with cocaine it would be useful. But if you are not planning to do that, you just cannot learn anything there.

Most of the rhetoric around alcohol and pregnancy is about IQ and behavior problems. But binge drinking is also implicated in miscarriage in the first trimester and in premature birth later. What about light drinking? Is this a concern?

In the case of premature birth, the answer is no. You can see this in studies in both Denmark and Italy (among other places). In the Italian study, women who drank up to 1 drink per day were actually less likely to have premature babies than those who did not drink at all. As in the case of IQ, there is no evidence of a link between preterm birth and light drinking; if anything, it looks like it lowers the risk.[10]

The evidence on miscarriage in the first trimester is a bit more mixed. A review article from 2007 summarized a number of studies. Several suggested there was no relationship between light drinking (in their case, up to 1 drink a day) and miscarriage. There were studies that suggested a link in particular subgroups (like among smokers), but the review dismissed these as largely unreliable. They concluded that there was no strong evidence for (or against) a relationship between light drinking and miscarriage.[11]

Somewhat at odds with this, however, is a new study released in early 2012 that analyzed the behavior of almost 100,000 Danish women and found that even light drinking (2 or more drinks a week) was associated with an increased risk of miscarriage in the first trimester.[12] These effects were fairly large—twice the risk of miscarriage for women drinking 4 or more drinks a week relative to those who drank none. This study wasn't perfect; they were not able to control for nausea, which other studies have shown to be an important mitigating factor (women who are nauseous drink less, and nausea is a good sign about a healthy pregnancy—more on this in the discussion of coffee).[13] But it does perhaps argue for limiting alcohol consumption more in the first trimester.

I talked to many, many pregnant women while working on this book (it helped that seemingly every person I have ever met got pregnant within a year of me). Virtually no one asked about drinking more than a drink a day. But I did wonder, largely from an academic standpoint: where is the line? If 5 at a time is bad and 1 at a time is not, what about 2 or 3?

It turned out to be hard to answer this very precisely. For one thing, the range here is big—1½ drinks a day is presumably less bad than 4½. In addition, the speed of drinking matters, so it's not even clear how we would frame this comparison. Also, almost no pregnant women drink at this level, so the data is mushy (not a technical term, but a good description!).

Two studies in Australia showed little or no difference in behavior problems and early language delays among children of slightly heavier drinkers (more than 1 but fewer than 5 drinks per day). [14, 15] So that's encouraging if you do want to drink that much. But other reasonable studies—one in France and one in Seattle—found decreased mental and physical development among young children of women who had 3 or more drinks per day. [16, 17]

There is also some evidence (from large-scale studies in Denmark and Italy) that drinking at this heavier level has short-term consequences such as stunted fetal growth and preterm labor.[18]

The mixed results and wide range of drinking behaviors in this category make it pretty hard to draw conclusions. However, especially at the higher levels of drinking in this range (say, 3 or more drinks per day), we start to see some evidence that this behavior might be risky. To be safe—to be cautious—I would argue that it seems best to stay at the lower end of this range, or out of it all together.

The bottom line is that the evidence overwhelmingly shows that light drinking is fine. In fact, there is virtually *no* evidence that drinking a glass of wine a day has negative impacts on pregnancy or child outcomes. Of course, this is a little sensitive to timing—7 drinks a week does not mean 7 shots of vodka in an hour on a Saturday night. Both the data and the science suggest that speed of drinking, and whether you are eating at the same time, matters. It's not that complicated: drink like a European adult, not like a fraternity brother.

In doing research for this book, I found the strength of the evidence in this case extremely surprising given the rhetoric around drinking during pregnancy in the United States. Many women I know seem unsure about having even a glass of wine at Christmas or on their anniversary, let alone having a few drinks a week. Yet there seems to be absolutely no reason for anything even close to these draconian restrictions. I am sure we can all see the case for wanting to stay well inside the danger zone, but drawing the line at any drinking at all seems, frankly, ridiculous.

One phrase I kept coming across was "no amount of alcohol has been proven safe." The implication, I suppose, is that we know that there exists a level of drinking that is bad, so we should assume all other levels are bad until proven otherwise. This seemed to me to have two problems.

First, too much anything can be bad. Tylenol overdose can lead to liver failure. In an extreme, even too much carrot juice would overdose you on Vitamin A. And yet Tylenol is routinely suggested to and taken by pregnant women, and no one would suggest limiting carrot juice.

Second, the statement that occasional drinking has not been proven safe could be applied to virtually anything in pregnancy. To Tylenol, yes, but also to many components of your prenatal vitamins, to coffee, and on and on. If what we require as proof is a large scale randomized trial, then it's right to say that alcohol hasn't been proven safe. But this would hold to a very different standard than most other behaviors. In fact, the type of evidence that leads to the argument that light drinking is not harmful is the same as the evidence that causes us to think heavier drinking is.

I drank the occasional glass of wine in the first trimester (I had one at that economist cocktail party, for example). I probably would have had more if it hadn't taken me the whole three months to finish this literature review. The rest of the time I had, perhaps, ½ glass 3 or 4 times a week. I rarely felt the desire for more than that. I liked the routine, a small drink at the end of the day with dinner, and ½ glass covered that. I took to heart the conclusion that a small amount at a time is the way to go. The one time I accidentally ordered half a liter of beer (who knew that wheat beers come in such large glasses?) I gave half to Jesse. That was almost certainly overcautious, but the pregnancy police were lurking.

The Bottom Line

- There is no good evidence that light drinking during pregnancy negatively impacts your baby. This means:

- Up to 1 drink a day in the second and third trimesters.

- 1 to 2 drinks a week in the first trimester.

- Speed matters: no vodka shots!

- Heavier drinking has negative impacts, especially in the range of four or five drinks at a time. This should be avoided.

Caffeine

I love coffee. After Penelope arrived this intensified with the sleep deprivation, of course, but even before I got pregnant I looked forward to a cup (or 2) with breakfast, a midmorning coffee break, and maybe a cup in the midafternoon as well. If you add it all together, I was up to 3 to 4 cups a day, depending on the day. This might seem like a lot (the average American consumes a bit less, more like three cups), but it's nothing relative to my caffeine habits in high school. Back then I could easily put away 2 or 3 cups after 9:00 P.M. with little impact on my sleep. The fact that I stick to decaf after 4:45 P.M. is among my strongest signals that I'm not 16 anymore!

With this background, the idea of giving up caffeine altogether during pregnancy was almost unthinkable. Of course, if it was important for Penelope I'd have done almost anything. But this was definitely a time when I hoped the evidence would come out a particular way.

My OB said some coffee was fine, but I should stick to less than 2 cups (again, that's an 8-ounce cup). I thought I could do that, although it definitely meant some limits, but then a friend told me her OB said no amount of coffee was acceptable, which is also what the *Mayo Clinic Guide to a Healthy Pregnancy* said. Was this the one time that my OB was actually not cautious *enough*?

The big concern with caffeine and pregnancy is that it might lead to higher rates of miscarriage. Caffeine can cross the placenta, and it's not clear how the fetus processes it. In addition, researchers have speculated that caffeine can inhibit fetal development by limiting blood flow to the placenta.

This is a case where the biological story on its own is not very compelling; although there is speculation about these effects, they have not been proven. What has been shown in a well-controlled way is that very high doses of caffeine do cause miscarriage in mice and rats. But these doses are much, much higher than what people consume. In order to produce pregnancy problems in rats, researchers require something like 250 milligrams of caffeine per kilogram per day. Translated to a human of 150 pounds? That's a bit more than 60 cups of coffee per day.[19] I challenge you to even find the time to drink that much!

To understand the impact of normal amounts of coffee in people, it's more helpful to look at studies of people. In the end, the challenges of drawing conclusions here are very similar to the challenges in the case of alcohol. Randomized experiments are difficult or impossible, and women who drink coffee tend to be different from those who don't.

Studies of the impact of caffeine on miscarriage have another problem, one that makes caffeine even harder to study than alcohol: nausea. Nausea is an unpleasant part of early pregnancy, one that most women experience. But (more on this later) it's also a really good sign about the health of the pregnancy. Women who experience nausea in early pregnancy are less likely to miscarry (it is not clear why this is the case; nausea may reflect hormone levels, but that's just speculation).

Why is this a problem? Consider this: my morning routine while *not* in the first trimester of pregnancy is to wake up, come downstairs, and turn on the coffee pot. I often have a cup before breakfast, on an empty stomach. Early in pregnancy this idea was, frankly, revolting. I would come downstairs and, instead of coffee, have a glass of club soda with lemon. I could occasionally bring myself to have a cup of coffee in the late afternoon, but only on especially good days. Talking with other women, it sounds like this is pretty typical.

We *know* that nausea is a sign of a healthy pregnancy. At the same time, it also causes women to avoid coffee. But this means that women who drink a lot of coffee are probably those who are *not* experiencing nausea. These women are more likely to miscarry. But you might be wrong to conclude that coffee causes miscarriage; it may well be that lack of nausea causes *both* miscarriage and coffee drinking.

This problem is pervasive throughout the studies we talk about here. Researchers try to "adjust" for this—asking women whether they experienced any nausea, for example—but this is hard to do. Nausea isn't a yes-or-no thing—some people are a little nauseated and some are a lot. The more sick you are, the better the sign about the pregnancy. Really, fully adjusting for this is basically impossible.

So, should we just give up and assume we can't draw any conclusions? Thankfully, that's probably not necessary. Even with this nausea issue, many studies suggest that in moderation there is no strong link between caffeine and miscarriage. Because we know the nausea issue will lead us to condemn coffee too quickly, this is especially reassuring.

But trying to figure out the impact of a lot of coffee (say, more than 4 cups a day) is a bit harder. There is some link with miscarriage, although, again, it may just be the nausea. You'll have to draw your own conclusions.

Up to 4 Cups Per Day

I started out trying to support my 3- to 4-cup-per-day coffee habit. I realized I probably got a bit more caffeine from other sources— say, soda or chocolate—but the caffeine content of everything other than coffee is really low (see box).

Perhaps my favorite study of this question is a recent one from Maryland published in 2010. The researchers followed a group of women starting when they tried to get pregnant. They collected daily diaries of their diets, including caffeine. By collecting the data every day, they didn't have to worry about the women forgetting how much coffee they had, and because they followed them from conception, they captured even early miscarriages. The women in this study had fairly normal caffeine consumption, with 75 percent of them having 3 cups or fewer of coffee per day.

This study found no relationship between caffeine and miscarriage. The big drawback, however, is the sample size: with data on only 66 pregnant women means this study is suggestive but not conclusive.[20]

But bigger studies often reached similar conclusions. Consider one covering about 2,400 women published in the journal *Epidemiology* in 2008.[21] Women enrolled in the study either while they were trying to get pregnant or at their first prenatal visit. Information on coffee consumption was collected at 16 weeks of pregnancy, and miscarriage was recorded up to 20 weeks.

A Caffeine Primer[22]

Caffeine content varies a lot, and across coffee brands in particular. Here's a little primer for some of the sources you might use most commonly:

- Starbucks brewed coffee, 8 oz.: 165 mg

- McDonald's brewed coffee, 8 oz.: 100 mg

- Starbucks latte, 16 oz.: 150 mg

- Black tea, 8 oz.: 14–61 mg, depending on the strength

- Green tea, 8 oz.: 24–40 mg, depending on the strength

- Coca-Cola, 12 oz.: 35 mg

- Mountain Dew, 12 oz.: 50 mg

You can see the results in the graph. Among the women who reported drinking no coffee, the miscarriage rate was about 10 percent. Women who consumed ½ cup to 2 cups a day had a slightly higher rate, but this difference is small. It's also not *statistically significant*. This means that it is likely that this is just random variation across groups, and not due to differences in coffee intake. Women who consumed even more coffee (more than 2 cups a day and more than 3½ cups a day) had, if anything, lower rates of miscarriage than those who consumed none (this difference is also not statistically significant).

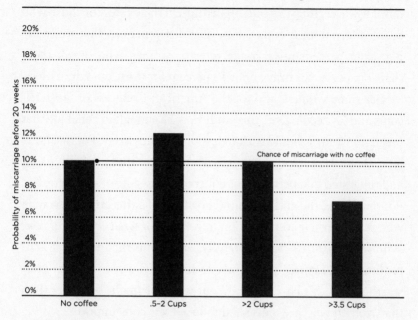

Coffee Drinking and Miscarriage

This study shows no evidence that miscarriage is associated with higher coffee consumption. The results remained true when they adjusted for differences across women in smoking, alcohol drinking, weight, and age. This isn't the only study to come to this conclusion—one in Denmark with almost 100,000 women similarly found no impacts of up to 3 cups of coffee a day.[23]

Having said this, not every study is so encouraging. Around the same time this 2008 study came out, a similar study was released in California. The study design was very close: researchers recruited women early in pregnancy, interviewed them about how much coffee they drank, and measured miscarriage up to 20 weeks. However, despite the similar design, the researchers came to somewhat different conclusions.[24]

This study differentiated among women who drank no coffee, those who drank less than 200 milligrams of coffee a day (2 cups), and those who drank more than that. The first thing to say is that the researchers found no difference in miscarriage rates between women who drank no coffee and those who drank up to 2 cups a day. However, they did find higher miscarriage rates for those who drank more than 2 cups a day. The differences in this study are big: a 25 percent miscarriage rate for women who drank more than 2 cups, versus only about 13 percent for those who drank less.

For some women, and for the American Congress of Obstetricians and Gynecologists, this study may be enough to conclude that pregnant women should stick to less than 2 cups a day. For me, however, there were enough aspects of the study that gave me pause and suggested that perhaps this is just the nausea story all over again. For one thing, the authors found no effect of coffee among women who reduced their consumption, *regardless of what their final consumption level was.* Taken literally, this means that it doesn't matter how much coffee you drink, as long as you reduce from your starting level. It's hard to figure out why this might be, other than that women who are nauseated reduce their consumption.

The authors are aware of the issue of nausea, and in some of their analyses they adjust for a yes/no question about nausea. The problem is that this doesn't go far enough. If asked in this study, I would say yes to nausea: I felt a little off for some of the first trimester, and I even vomited once. But I wasn't so sick that I avoided coffee completely; I just cut down. My friend Jane would also say yes; she was vomiting every day, multiple times a day, for at least 6 weeks. The idea that she would have coffee at all was ridiculous.

The degree of nausea varies a lot. The association between nausea and miscarriage means that the sicker you feel, the better. But the sicker you are, the less coffee you want. To really do a good job adjusting for this, you'd need to know much more about how sick people were. This is very difficult; it's not so much a criticism of this particular study as a comment on the whole research program. As one review article concludes, it's basically impossible to separate caffeine and nausea, and it's possible, even likely, that *all* evidence of a caffeine-miscarriage link is due to this issue.[25]

As I poked around this research, there were a few other things that made me think the nausea story might be quite important. One was that other common sources of caffeine—tea and cola— are less consistently linked with miscarriage.[26] These contain caffeine (although less than coffee), but tend to be easier on the stomach, so the confounding relationship with nausea is limited. If caffeine was really a problem independent of nausea, I would have expected coffee and tea to have similar impacts.

I also found one clever study that showed that decaffeinated coffee was as strongly linked to miscarriage as caffeinated coffee. Decaf coffee has the same nausea problem, but no caffeine. If the real problem was caffeine, why would decaf coffee matter? It didn't *prove* the case, but it was pretty suggestive.[27]

I ultimately concluded that the weight of the evidence didn't support limiting my consumption very much. I decided the 3 to 4 cups a day I was having was fine. It's possible you will read this evidence and decide that you would like to stay under 2 cups. There's no reason to have less than that if you feel up to it.

After the first trimester, fears about miscarriage decline. The remaining concern with caffeine is that it might be linked to slow fetal growth or preterm birth, both of which are serious complications.

I was really hoping there would be compelling evidence on this, because the one thing that happened as I got more and more pregnant was a dramatic increase in questions about whether it was okay for me to have coffee. These questions usually occurred in the faculty lounge at work as I was waiting for my latte. I think people were typically quite sorry they asked, given the amount of information I threw at them. But I was well prepared: this is a case in which the evidence is much better.

The evidence is better for the simple reason that there is at least one randomized controlled trial (I guess it's not impossible to get this by an ethical review board, just difficult). Researchers in Denmark recruited 1,207 pregnant women who were coffee drinkers (at least 3 cups a day). They were asked to be in the study before 20 weeks of pregnancy, and the researchers recorded the birth weight of their babies and whether they were premature.[28]

Now here is the experiment: women were given free instant coffee. Half of them were given free *caffeinated* instant coffee, and half were given free *decaffeinated* instant coffee. The women did not know which type of coffee they received (the boxes looked the same). They were asked to replace their usual coffee with the instant coffee from the study.

So what happened? The women given the caffeinated instant coffee consumed a lot more caffeine (not surprising!). They consumed about 200 milligrams more of caffeine than the decaf group. In all other ways these women looked the same (same age, same chance of being a smoker, and so on). Because they were similar in other ways, any differences the researchers observed between the groups could be attributed to the differences in coffee intake. On the other hand, if they did *not* observe any differences, they could conclude that giving people more caffeine did not impact their babies.

In fact, this "lack of effect" is exactly what they found. Even though the caffeinated-coffee group drank a lot more caffeine, their babies looked exactly the same. The table below shows information about the children of women in this study.

	Children of Women Getting Decaffeinated Instant Coffee	Children of Women Getting Caffeinated Instant Coffee
Birth Weight	7 pounds, 12 ounces	7 pounds, 12.8 ounces
Length at Birth	20.4 inches	20.5 inches
Gestational Age at Birth	279.3 days	280.2 days
Head Circumference	13.8 inches	13.8 inches

The caffeinated-coffee women had babies of the same weight and length after the same number of days of gestation, and with the same head size. Other, nonrandomized studies have reached similar conclusions.[29]

More Than 4 Cups Per Day (Wow!)

I'm probably on the high end of coffee consumption, but I'm not at the maximum. For at least some people, having 6, 7, or 8 cups of coffee a day is not unusual. A couple of those Dunkin' Donuts extra-large coffees and you are getting close to that. If you are in that group, is there any reason to cut down?

The first thing to note is that studies of women at this higher level of consumption are, if anything, even more subject to the concerns about nausea. If you are feeling at all nauseous, at any time of the day, you are probably not having 8 cups of coffee. Perhaps for this reason—or, perhaps, because too much coffee really is a problem—studies are more consistent at showing a link between very high caffeine intake and miscarriage. One study in Denmark included almost 100,000 women and focused on late miscarriage, after 16 weeks of pregnancy.[30] Miscarriage in this period is not very common, so the overall numbers in the study are small.

Nevertheless, they found higher miscarriage rates for women who drank 8 or more cups of coffee a day versus those who avoided it all together: 1.9 percent of women in the high-caffeine group miscarried, versus 1.2 percent in the low-caffeine group.*

A second study, this one from Sweden and published in the

---

* These figures take the miscarriage rate for 0 cups as the baseline, and calculate the higher-intake groups by multiplying this baseline by the adjusted hazard ratio. You can read this as saying: if the group drinking 8 cups of coffee was similar on all the other variables to the 0 cups group, their miscarriage rate would be 1.9 percent, versus 1.2 percent in the 0 cups group.

prestigious *New England Journal of Medicine,* also included some
women with these very high rates of coffee intake (I surmise that
my northern European ancestors drank more coffee than most).[31]
In this case, the researchers considered earlier miscarriage (between
6 and 12 weeks). The study began with a sample of around 550
women who were known to have had a miscarriage between 6 and
12 weeks, plus roughly 1,000 similar women who were pregnant
around the same time but *did not* have a miscarriage.

This study found an increased risk of miscarriage at high levels of caffeine consumption. Relative to those women who drank
1 cup or less per day, women who drank more than 5 cups a day
were twice as likely to lose their baby.

Again, the specter of nausea raises its head, this time
in a slightly different way. The women who miscarried were interviewed *after* their loss, and asked about their coffee intake in the
last weeks of pregnancy. Even if they remembered correctly, this
poses a problem. Many miscarriages are "missed"—that is, the
fetus dies a week or two before the miscarriage becomes apparent. The death of the fetus often means the end of nausea. But
that means in the week or two before they learned they had a
miscarriage, these women would have been feeling better, and
possibly had more coffee.

In other words, maybe it wasn't the coffee that caused the miscarriage, but the miscarriage that caused the increase in coffee.

In my view, a reasonable person could see the case for reducing caffeine intake, and a similarly reasonable person could conclude that the results are probably all driven by differences in
nausea and therefore continue on as before.

The Bottom Line

- In moderation, coffee is fine.

- All evidence supports having up to 2 cups.

- Much of the evidence supports having 3 to 4 cups.

- Evidence on more than 4 cups a day is mixed; some links are seen with miscarriage, but it is possible that they are all due to the effects of nausea.

Tobacco

It seems safe to say that most women drink alcohol and consume caffeine when not pregnant and that both substances are generally accepted to be safe outside of pregnancy (in some moderation; not while driving; etc). In contrast, tobacco is not recommended to anyone at any time.

If you smoke, your doctor has presumably encouraged you to quit. But quitting is hard, and most smokers have tried at one time or another. The question in the case of pregnancy: is there any *extra* reason to quit while pregnant?

The answer is a resounding yes. Smoking, even in moderate amounts, is bad for your baby. Women who smoke are at a higher risk for preterm labor, problems with their placenta, and low-birth-weight babies. Further, the babies of women who smoke are at higher risk for SIDS (sudden infant death syndrome, sometimes called crib death). The good news is that quitting anytime during pregnancy mitigates these problems.

The exact science of why smoking matters is not completely clear, but we have some idea. Tobacco contains a number of chemicals, but the two important ones are nicotine and carbon monoxide. Both of these restrict oxygen to the fetus. Less oxygen means less growth. Additionally, the blood vessel constriction caused by nicotine exposure can damage the placenta, which is the source of many pregnancy complications.

We can see these complications directly. Consider a representative study that analyzed *all births* in Missouri between 1989 and 2005 (this amounted to more than 1 million babies).[32] The authors in this study simply looked at whether women said they smoked during pregnancy, and compared women who smoked to those who did not. The table below shows the chances of common pregnancy complications for smokers and nonsmokers.

Maternal Smoking Behavior and Pregnancy Complications

	% of Nonsmokers with This Complication	% of Smokers with This Complication
Anemia	1.39%	1.70%
Eclampsia	0.10%	0.09%
Placental Abruption	0.71%	1.27%
Placenta Previa	0.35%	0.48%
Baby Small for Gestational Age	7.47%	17.08%
Preterm Birth	10.55%	13.64%
Stillbirth	0.44%	0.61%

The complications included here are varied, some impacting the mother and some the baby. Women who smoke are more likely to be anemic, and are much more likely to have problems with the placenta and to have preterm births or stillbirths. The impacts on birth weight are huge: if you smoke you are more than twice as likely to have a baby who is very small.

With alcohol, there is an important difference between moderate drinking and very heavy drinking. Maybe moderate smoking is okay? No, it is not. The study in Missouri showed that women smoking 1 to 9 cigarettes a day had just has many extra complications as those smoking more than a pack.

Does it matter when during pregnancy you smoke? A study from the Netherlands published in 2008 looked at the timing of smoking.[33] These authors found that smoking later in pregnancy had the largest effects on birth weight. The graph below shows baby birth weight for women who smoked before 18 weeks and after 25 weeks of pregnancy.

Women who smoked more than 9 cigarettes a day after 25 weeks had babies about 7 ounces smaller than those who did not smoke; this is a 6 percent reduction in body weight! This means, among other things, that even if you smoke at the start of pregnancy, there are still huge benefits to quitting later on.

What may be particularly frightening is that risks to the baby do not seem to be limited to their time in the womb. A study in the United Kingdom described differences in the risk of SIDS in

Impact of Smoking on Birth Weight, by Timing of Smoking:
Data from the Netherlands

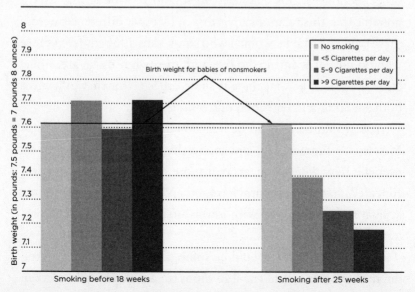

children of mothers who smoked and those who did not.[34] Children of mothers who smoked 1 to 9 cigarettes a day during pregnancy were more than 4 times as likely to die of SIDS as those whose mothers did not smoke. Children of mothers who smoked 20 or more cigarettes a day were almost 9 times as likely to die. Here is another way to look at it: 86 percent of SIDS deaths in England were among children of mothers who smoked.

It turns out that it is not just Mom's smoking that matters. Secondhand smoke exposure (for example, from fathers or grandparents) also leads to many of the same negative outcomes. A 2010 review article found that babies of mothers who were exposed to secondhand smoke during pregnancy were about 2 ounces lighter at birth than babies who were not.[35] It's worth saying that the women in these studies were exposed to a lot of smoke, like the amount that would come from living with a husband who smokes. Very occasional contact (a night in a restaurant with smokers, or walking by someone smoking on the street) is not a big deal.

So it looks like smoking is dangerous. But if you have read the other sections of this chapter, you should be wondering: isn't it possible that this relationship is driven by other differences across these women? Maybe women who smoke are different from those who do not, or women who live with men who smoke are different. Or could it be that there is some other factor that influences both smoking and bad child outcomes?

You would be right to be concerned. Take that first study in Missouri.[36] Women who smoked in that study were different on average: they were younger, had more other children, were less educated, had less prenatal care, etc. Many of these factors are known to be associated with lower-birth-weight babies and preterm delivery.

As usual, our ideal would be some randomized evidence. You might think this would run into the same problems as the alcohol and coffee cases—who is going to let you experiment with forcing people to smoke? However, it turns out that precisely *because* people are convinced that smoking is bad, and because it is hard to stop, there are randomized trials that do exactly the opposite: encourage women to quit smoking.

Typically, these studies take a group of pregnant smokers and randomly assign half of them to some treatment that will hopefully reduce their smoking. If some of the women do quit smoking, we can learn about the impacts of smoking by comparing their babies with the babies of women in the control groups.

A 2008 review article summarized 64 studies just like this,[37] 16 of which also collected information on the babies. One thing we learn is that it's really hard to quit smoking: of these 16 trials, only 5 actually got a significant number of women to quit. But among those studies we see benefits for the baby: women who were encouraged to quit had babies who were about 2 ounces heavier.

This may not seem like a lot, but consider this: even the treatments that worked had really tiny effects. On average, about 90 percent of women who were in the control group continued to smoke, along with 80 percent of those who were in the encouraged-to-quit group. The impact of not smoking must be very large if we can see differences in average birth weight across the two groups even with such small differences in the number of smokers. For at least one of the studies included in this review, a follow-up study rescaled these estimates to calculate the impact of completely quitting smoking on birth weight. They estimated an impact of 14 ounces, or almost a full pound!

The impacts on preterm birth are even more striking. Despite the small changes in smoking rates, the studies found that women who were encouraged to quit had a 28 percent decrease in the chance of preterm birth.

Here is an example of a case where the medical recommendation is spot-on: if you are smoking when you get pregnant or are trying to get pregnant, this is yet another reason to quit. Smoking is already bad for you, and it's really bad for your fetus. Randomized trials show that quitting smoking has big benefits. The good news is that you can experience these benefits anytime. There's no evidence that smoking before pregnancy creates problems. Even quitting partway through is better than continuing.[38]

A final note: the best option is to quit smoking cold turkey as soon as you find out you are pregnant, or, ideally, before. But what if you can't just stop, or can't stop without help? More specifically, is it a good idea to try nicotine replacement therapy (gum, patches, etc.)?

There are, in fact, a number of randomized controlled trials of NRTs, but the evidence is not conclusive. The main problem is that most of these studies have no impact on smoking rates: women do not seem to stop smoking when given NRTs. This makes it hard to figure out the impact on their babies.[39] There is positive evidence from at least one study in which women offered nicotine gum decreased the number of cigarettes they smoked. This study found that babies born to the women offered the gum had birth weights an average of 11 ounces larger than women who were not offered the gum. This is promising, but not conclusive. As these therapies require a prescription, talking to your doctor is a must, and may provide better guidance about the value of these interventions for you personally.[40]

The Bottom Line

Smoking during pregnancy is dangerous for your baby.

. . .

Miscarriage Fears

n trying to learn the truth about alcohol and, in particular, caffeine, it was hard to avoid discussion of miscarriage. Increased risk of miscarriage is the major (overstated) concern about excess caffeine consumption. And it was something I thought about—worried about—a lot. When I first got the positive pregnancy test I was worried it would turn out to be a false alarm once I checked with the doctor. Then, once she confirmed the pregnancy, I was worried it wouldn't proceed normally.

In my seventh week I went to the doctor (already my third visit) for an early ultrasound. Early ultrasounds like this can be used for very accurate pregnancy dating. Because the fetal growth is so fast early on in pregnancy, a good ultrasound can detect the difference between a pregnancy that is, for example, 6 weeks and 4 days along versus 6 weeks and 6 days.

If things are developing normally, this ultrasound can be pretty amazing. You will almost certainly see some evidence of a baby by this point—an actual embryo, or at least evidence that the egg is implanted. If you are far enough along, you may actually hear (or, more likely, "see") evidence of a heartbeat on the ultrasound. I remember this ultrasound and the moment Penelope was born as the two times I realized nothing would ever be quite the same again.

Of course I was excited about this ultrasound, but I was also nervous. The flip side of being able to see if things are developing normally is that doctors can also see at this point if there is a problem. If you have an ectopic pregnancy, this is probably when you would find out. They may also see that the embryo is simply not developing, a likely sign that you will miscarry.

Seeing that all was well reassured me for a moment, but it was really just a moment. If anything, knowing that there was something to lose made me even more nervous about miscarriage.

There wasn't anything I could do—I knew that. It is estimated that 90 percent of miscarriages in the first trimester are a result of chromosomal problems. All my research thus far had suggested that, other than not smoking, there wasn't much I could do to prevent this from happening. And yet I still wanted to know the risks—to have some concrete numbers.

I knew I wasn't alone in this. One morning shortly after Penelope was born, I woke up to a text from my best friend, who had just recently found out she was expecting: "For peace of mind, do you have a chart on miscarriage rates by week for a healthy 31 year old? Thanks! Trish."

I realized that not only is there not some easily accessible chart I could point Tricia to, it was hard even to get a sense of the magnitude of the miscarriage risk from popular discussion. We all know that there is some risk of pregnancy loss in the first trimester, and that it is lower after 12 weeks. But how high, and how much lower?

It is convention, in the United States at least, to wait until the end of the first trimester to tell people about a pregnancy; one reason for this is that this is the time after which the highest risk of miscarriage has past. Given the seriousness with which people seem to adhere to this convention, you would not be faulted for thinking that there is some sharp change in the miscarriage risk at 12 or 13 weeks. In fact, I briefly fell victim to this as well, trying to calculate whether 12 or 13.33 weeks was actually the first "trimester." Of course, biology doesn't really work in a sharp way like this. Miscarriage risk falls as your pregnancy progresses, but there is no special drop down at 12 weeks.

The twelve-week rule seems to be more of a social norm than anything else. Because this is around the time most women start to show, at least a bit, that may have contributed to the convention. Certainly your doctor is unlikely to have much to say about this—when you tell your colleagues about a baby isn't much of a medical decision! Although there isn't anything special about 12 weeks, the probability of miscarriage does decrease over the course of the pregnancy.

Before 5 or so weeks, a pregnancy is considered *chemical*, not *clinical* (just a reminder: pregnancy is counted from the first day of your last period, so 5 weeks is 1 week past your missed period). This is the period of time when you can detect the pregnancy with a test but you wouldn't yet see it on an ultrasound. Many pregnancies are lost in this period; perhaps as many as half. I spoke a bit about this in the chapter on conception. It is only recently that pregnancy tests have been able to pick up evidence of a pregnancy this early.

After 6 weeks, when your doctors can see evidence of your pregnancy on an ultrasound (if they are looking), the pregnancy is clinical. This is around the time most women have their first prenatal visit. Assuming that things look as they should at this first visit, miscarriage rates after that are low to moderate, and they decrease as the pregnancy progresses. The easiest way to see the numbers is by looking at studies that follow women whose first prenatal visits came at different points in their pregnancies. Researchers can then look at how many women miscarry among those with a normal visit at 6 weeks, how many miscarry among those with a normal visit at 7 weeks, and so on. In this way they can map out the miscarriage risk by week of pregnancy.

The graph below is an answer to Tricia's question. It shows her the miscarriage risk by week of pregnancy, averaging across three similar studies.[1]

If you are seen at 6 weeks and things look normal, what is the overall chance that you will have a miscarriage? The data suggests about 11 percent. If you are seen later, say, at 8 weeks, and things look normal at that point, then the chance of miscarriage is lower, about 6 percent. By the eleventh week, it has dropped to less than 2 percent.

These rates are just an average. There are a number of factors that may raise or lower your personal risk relative to the average individual. One factor is a previous history of miscarriage: having had one miscarriage, you are somewhat more likely to have another. A study in England showed that the chance of first-trimester miscarriage was around 4 to 5 percent for first pregnan-

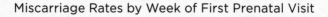

Miscarriage Rates by Week of First Prenatal Visit

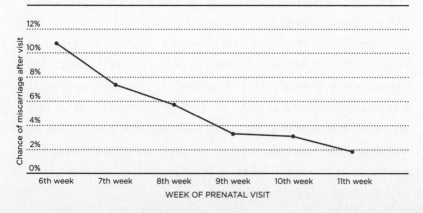

cies or women with a previous successful pregnancy. But for those
with a previous miscarriage, it was around 25 percent.[2] This may
seem scary, but it is important to remember that most women
who miscarry—the vast majority—go on to have successful
pregnancies.

A second factor is age. Older women are more likely to miscarry (this is likely related to a higher rate of chromosomal problems). These effects are large. In one study the miscarriage rate
was 4.4 percent for women under 20, 6.7 percent for women 20
to 35, and almost 19 percent for women over 35.[3] Relatedly, pregnancies achieved via IVF seem also to be more likely to end in
miscarriage. One large study reported a miscarriage rate of 30
percent for IVF pregnancies, versus 19 percent for those achieved
naturally.[4]

In addition to these prepregnancy risk factors, there are a couple of symptoms during early pregnancy that correlate with miscarriage. One is vaginal bleeding. Bleeding is very common in the
first trimester, and most of the time is not something to worry
about. However, it does indicate a slightly higher risk of miscarriage: in one study, 13 percent of women with bleeding ended up
miscarrying, versus only 4.2 percent of women without.[5] A second is *lack of* nausea. Women who are *not* nauseous are more
likely to miscarry than those who are.

You might wonder if there is something you can do (other
than getting pregnant at 20 rather than at 35!). The answer is
probably not. As most pregnancy losses at this point are due to
chromosomal problems and those are determined at fertilization,
it is out of your control.[6] For a small number of women, low levels
of progesterone may contribute to early miscarriage; this can
sometimes be corrected with a progesterone supplement. How
important this is and the right solution are of some debate in the
medical literature. If you have had several miscarriages, it is
something your doctor might consider.

The graph above, which I sent Tricia, stops at 11 weeks. (Happily, she didn't need it: at 38 weeks and 6 days she delivered a healthy baby boy.) In the second trimester miscarriage is less common, but it does happen. Most studies put the overall risk of fetal loss after 12 weeks at 1 to 2 percent.[7] One very large study, of almost 300,000 women, demonstrated miscarriage rates of as low as 0.6 percent after 15 weeks.[8] These figures were a bit higher for older women, just as in the case of first-trimester miscarriage, but still quite low.

Amazingly, by 22 or 23 weeks some babies can actually survive outside the womb (although this is rare and usually comes with serious disabilities). Then you're in the range of preterm birth, which we will leave to a later chapter.

The Bottom Line

- Around 10 to 15 percent of pregnancies that are developing normally at 6 weeks will end in miscarriage. This rate declines quickly over the first trimester, and falls to around 1 to 2 percent by 11 or 12 weeks.

- Older age and previous miscarriage increase your risk.

Beware of Deli Meats!

As soon as I got back from my conference, I headed to my doctor's office for a blood test to confirm that I was pregnant (I was). As I was leaving I was handed a list of do's and don'ts. The limits on alcohol, caffeine, and tobacco were there, of course. But most of the list involved food. I couldn't believe how many foods were off-limits: hot dogs, raw oysters, deli meats, lox, rare steak, sushi, and on and on. For a while I carried the list around, worried I'd forget something.

The one that really irked me was tuna. Normally, I'd say I have an average level of interest in tuna-fish sandwiches. When I got pregnant, however, I developed what can only be described as an insatiable craving for them. Every day at the cafeteria I stared longingly at the sandwich counter before settling on something less exciting. I allowed myself about one tuna sandwich a week, following my OB's advice to "limit" tuna consumption. I couldn't wait until the baby was out, when I would eat tuna melts for breakfast, lunch, and dinner for a week. Of course, once Penelope was born I no longer had any interest in tuna.

More or less every mother I know has this kind of story about one of the pregnancy food restrictions. Jane was constantly talking about Italian subs (forbidden due to restrictions on deli meats). Another friend missed sushi so much that she had someone lined up to bring her some at the hospital as soon as her daughter was born; of course, like my experience, as soon as the baby was out, her craving was gone as well.

As I stared longingly at the tuna salad, or picked at my vegetable "sushi" while everyone else enjoyed a spicy salmon roll, Jesse would constantly question the restrictions. "What's the big deal?" he would say, waving a wasabi-coated piece of raw fish in front of me. "You eat this stuff normally and it doesn't make you sick; why avoid it now?" And maybe it was just the cravings, but I started to wonder, was he right? Was I any more likely to get food poisoning while pregnant? And was there any real added danger if I did?

I also started to wonder if all the food restrictions were created equal. Were oysters worse than swordfish? Were they even off-limits for the same reason? And, as usual, the restrictions were inconsistent. I asked my doctor at one point about prosciutto, which I thought was pretty clearly a deli meat. She looked at me like I was crazy and asked, "Why would you think that's a problem?" Apparently not all meats that go into deli sandwiches actually count as deli meats. But the lists I found on the Internet *did* restrict prosciutto. I maintain that it was reasonable to be confused.

I realized that I needed something more organized—some kind of framework. Rather than just a list of foods that are good or not so good, I needed to understand the more general reason why some foods were restricted. If I had this, I could then figure out which were really bad, and which were only kind of bad. I would also be in a better position to think about things like prosciutto. If I knew the problem with deli meats, I could figure out if prosciutto should count or not.

The vast majority of pregnancy food restrictions arise from

concerns about food contamination. If you undercook a burger, and the meat comes from a meat processing plant that is also home to a bacteria like E. coli, you will very likely be sorry the next day. If you use a raw egg in your Caesar dressing and the chicken that laid it had salmonella, you're exposed to the bacteria and run the risk of illness. I will stop here, but I'll say that I don't recommend immersing yourself in food safety issues unless you want to spend a week as a paranoid germaphobe.

But these things are true *regardless* of pregnancy. No doctor was pressuring Jesse to avoid a medium-rare burger, even though there was always the possibility that he could get sick as well.

I was already taking normal precautions about food. No gas station sushi, for example. Knowing that food could make me sick didn't really tell me whether I should be more cautious during pregnancy. It seemed clear that there were two questions: If I ate the same way I normally did, was I more likely to get sick while pregnant? And if I did get sick, was there any risk to the baby?

The answer wasn't the same for every restricted food: not all food-borne bacteria are created equal. The table below lists the common food restrictions during pregnancy (minus my beloved tuna, which is restricted for mercury reasons and I'll talk about that later). For each food, you can also see the food safety issue:

Pregnancy Off-limits Food List

- Raw eggs (salmonella)

- Raw fish (salmonella, campylobacter)

- Raw shellfish (salmonella, campylobacter, toxoplasmosis)

continued

- Unwashed vegetables and fruits (toxoplasmosis, E. coli)

- Raw/rare meat and poultry (salmonella, toxoplasmosis, campylobacter, E. coli)

- Smoked fish (Listeria)

- Pâté (Listeria)

- Unpasteurized (raw) milk (Listeria, campylobacter)

- Raw milk soft cheese (Listeria)

- Deli meats (Listeria)

Let's start with an obvious point: some of these foods are not that hard to avoid. Raw poultry, for example, would rarely be served except by accident. Raw eggs may be an occasional salad dressing ingredient, but avoiding them feels like a minor change. Similarly, unwashed vegetables can be easily avoided by washing them, which hopefully you are doing anyway.

But other risky foods are more common and more delicious: a rare steak, a turkey sandwich, a nice raw-milk brie. There are five types of infection that are possible from these foods: salmonella, E. coli, campylobacter, Listeria, and toxoplasmosis (actually caused by a parasite, not a bacteria). In fact, three of the five are really no worse during pregnancy than at any other time!

Salmonella, E. Coli, and Campylobacter: Proceed with *normal* caution. Salmonella and E. coli are by far the most common causes of food-borne illnesses. Campylobacter is similar in its effects, although less common. All three bacteria cause basic stomach-flu symptoms: diarrhea, nausea, and vomiting. Unless you are very lucky or have a stomach made of iron, you have probably been sickened by one of these before. It's unpleasant, sure. But illnesses from these causes are not especially more likely during pregnancy, nor do they typically directly affect the fetus.*

Beyond a little added caution, always a good idea even when not pregnant, things that are restricted due to these bugs shouldn't really be completely off your list during pregnancy. If we look at the list above, this means that raw fish and raw eggs should at least be back on a "sometimes" list (assuming you typically eat them). Eating raw eggs from a slightly postdated carton from 7-Eleven is probably best avoided. But by *everyone*, not just pregnant women.

I was excited to realize that Jesse had been right all along about sushi. I decided that I didn't need to be much more careful than before I was pregnant. I ate at my neighborhood sushi bar before, and I kept doing that. I did stop eating the sushi that they keep sitting around in the cooler at work, but largely because the idea of a stomach flu when I was already pretty uncomfortable was too much to bear!

I started to get greedy. Maybe there was no reason to worry about *any* of these bacteria. That turned out to be wrong: both toxoplasmosis and Listeria are particular pregnancy concerns.

Toxoplasmosis: Harmful but largely avoidable. If you have heard of this in the context of pregnancy, it was almost certainly related to cat litter, not food. Toxoplasmosis is caused by a parasite—toxoplasma gondii—and concerns about this parasite are the reason pregnant women are told to avoid cleaning the litter box. However, you are quite a bit more likely to get this from raw meat or unwashed vegetables than from cat litter (more on the feline source later). In nonpregnant people, toxoplasmosis infection is not usually an issue (it can cause flulike symptoms). The symptoms are similar during pregnancy. The big danger is that many people who are infected do not notice any symptoms at all; if you notice symptoms, you can be treated and reduce the

---

* There is actually one variant of the salmonella bacteria that can pass to the fetus, but it's not one that we have in the United States.

chance of passing the parasite to your baby. But if you don't notice them or the treatment doesn't work, the fetus can become infected.

If your fetus becomes infected with the parasite, it may develop what is called congenital toxoplasmosis. This affects about 1 in 1,500 babies.[1] The complications of congenital toxoplasmosis include mental retardation, blindness, and epilepsy. The severity varies widely and is related to the timing of infection: infection early in pregnancy is worse than later.

Avoiding toxoplasmosis is not that difficult. It comes primarily from undercooked meats, and possibly dried or cured meat (like prosciutto), although the latter is less common.[2] Based on a study in Europe, about 10 percent of toxoplasmosis cases could be avoided by washing vegetables and fruits well before eating them. Another third to a half could be avoided by not eating raw or very undercooked meat. About a third of cases are of unknown origin. This makes a good case for washing your veggies and avoiding raw and undercooked meat, which would dramatically limit your exposure.

There is one caveat to this. It is possible that you already have toxoplasmosis. Many people (perhaps 25 percent of people in the United States)[3] carry this bacteria, having been infected sometime in the past—through a cat (if you clean a litter box), through eating or handling uncooked meat, or through gardening (because animals, like cats, poop in the soil). If you have already had this infection, *there is no risk to your baby.* Having had this in the past is not a problem, and you cannot be reinfected. If you already carry the parasite, you are in the clear. If you are curious, your doctor can test for this at the start of pregnancy.

I actually have a cat, and I did as a child as well, so it is possible that I have already been exposed to this. But I wasn't tested, and I did avoid rare meat. This was frequently depressing. Jesse's one and only contribution to cooking in the household is his use of the grill, and he makes an excellent steak. I like mine medium rare.

During pregnancy, Jesse would cook mine to a dry hunk of charcoal while he continued to enjoy his very rare. Once I suggested he should eat his well done in solidarity. That got a good laugh.

Listeria: Harmful and hard to avoid. Listeria in pregnancy is very dangerous. Listeria infection begins with standard stomach-flu symptoms but typically gets worse, including chills and muscle aches. It can be fatal even in healthy adults, and pregnant women are much more susceptible: up to a third of all Listeria infections are in pregnant women. Thankfully, Listeria is not that common: about one in eight thousand pregnancies a year are affected.[4]

But if you are infected, the consequences are scary. Miscarriage, preterm birth, or stillbirth are common outcomes, occurring in between 10 and 50 percent of pregnant women who are infected.[5] Complications for surviving infants include meningitis, neurological problems, and other complications from premature delivery. Recent research in guinea pigs has suggested that this may occur because the placenta becomes infected and then continually reinfects the mother; expelling the placenta (and the baby) may be the body's natural protective response.[6] Regardless of why it occurs, it's a devastating outcome and scary to contemplate.

There *is* reason to worry about Listeria. But I realized that I still didn't know enough to know how careful I should be about the actual *foods* on the Listeria list. Clearly it's a bad idea to go out and snack directly on some Listeria bacteria. But how important were these particular foods? How completely could I avoid these risks by following the food restrictions?

Think about two different scenarios.

Scenario 1: 95 percent of Listeria cases are caused by a single food—say, carrots—and 5 percent are caused by something unknown. If you want to avoid Listeria, you could therefore do pretty well by avoiding carrots—you drop your risk by 95 percent.

Scenario 2: only 5 percent of Listeria cases are caused by carrots, and 95 percent are caused by various other things that are hard to identify. It is still the case that carrots are the *most* common source of Listeria, but by eliminating carrots you avoid only about 5 percent of cases. You might still want to avoid carrots, but there is less reason to do so: it's just not as beneficial as it was in the scenario where carrots were responsible for 95 percent of Listeria cases.

To figure out which of these scenarios was correct—and what particular foods to avoid—I needed to figure out what foods were linked to Listeria and what share of the Listeria outbreaks each food accounted for. I thought it would be easiest to start with the last few big outbreaks.

This led me in a pretty odd direction.

The last two major outbreaks prior to my pregnancy were in celery (in 2010) and cantaloupes (in 2011). The cantaloupe outbreak was large, covered many states, and caused 29 deaths. In 2008 there was a large outbreak due to sprouts. When I was pregnant with my son in 2015 there was a large outbreak in ice cream. The last confirmed Listeria outbreak due to deli meats was back in 2005. A lot of these outbreaks seemed pretty random. There was no way to know beforehand that I should have avoided celery in October 2010.

Part of what makes this bacteria tricky is that it is very difficult to pin down the source of a Listeria infection. Between 2000 and 2008, the CDC was able to identify sources for only 262 of the estimated 24,000 cases. This is largely because the time between infection and illness can be as long as a month or even two. It's easy to identify the source of illness if the patient has to remember only what he or she ate yesterday, but recalling all food consumption in the past three or four weeks will challenge most people.

There are, however, a couple of consistent causes of Listeria. Over the period from 1998 to 2008, there were 29 outbreaks that the CDC could identify sources for. In 17 percent of them, the culprit was queso fresco (a Mexican-style soft cheese often made from unpasteurized milk). Another 10 percent were traced to deli turkey. One general rule: Listeria grows well at refrigerator temperatures, so any food that has been sitting around a long time in the fridge should probably be avoided.

Ultimately, this is something you need to decide for yourself. The question is not whether Listeria infection is scary: it is. The question is what decisions you can make to avoid it. It would be difficult or impossible to avoid all foods that have caused a Listeria outbreak—not just deli turkey, but cantaloupes, sprouts, celery, taco salad, grilled chicken, and on and on. Even if you did avoid all these foods, Listeria could well show up in apples next, or pork chops. There's just no way to know.

The link with Mexican-style cheese seems especially strong to me, and I avoided it (easily, because I don't even know where I would find it). I also mostly avoided turkey, although I didn't extend the restriction to other deli meats. It seemed unfair to tar them with the same brush. My best estimate, based on the data, was that avoiding ham sandwiches would have lowered my risk of Listeria infection from 1 in 8,333 to 1 in 8,255. Would you want to do this? Maybe. Someone certainly could make a case for doing so. However, this change is really, really small. For me, it wasn't worth it.

In the end, I narrowed the restricted-food list down to just a few things.

Oster Updated Off-limits Food List

- Raw/rare meat and poultry (toxoplasmosis)

- Unwashed vegetables and fruits (toxoplasmosis)

- Queso fresco and other raw-milk cheeses (Listeria)

- Deli turkey (Listeria)

Of course, you might decide on something a bit different. You might, for example, want to add cantaloupe to the list.

A final note: what should you do if you do get sick? The somewhat good news is that, for both listeriosis and toxoplasmosis, early treatment can reduce (although not eliminate) the chance of transmission to your baby. If you are feeling sick, be more cautious than usual. Don't just ride it out and take some Imodium; at least *call* the doctor.

The Bottom Line

- Don't worry too much about sushi and raw eggs—they might carry bacteria, but these bacteria are no worse when you are pregnant than when you are not.

- Toxoplasmosis infection during pregnancy can be damaging to your baby. The risks are small, and you can cut your risk in half by thoroughly washing your vegetables and by not eating raw or rare meat.

- The most dangerous food-borne bacteria is Listeria. Unfortunately, a lot of sources of outbreaks are random: cantaloupes, celery, sprouts. Avoiding Listeria is very desirable, but may be difficult due to the random nature of the outbreaks. Based on past outbreaks, you would do well to avoid queso fresco and, probably, turkey sandwiches.

- The CDC has a very helpful general source for information about food outbreaks: http://www.cdc.gov/foodborneburden/index.html. If there is another cantaloupe-related outbreak, you'll probably hear about it there first!

- If you do get sick, call your doctor.

When I finally emerged from the unappetizing world of food contamination, I realized I still didn't have the answer to my main question: could I have a tuna sandwich? Tuna fell into the second group of restricted foods: high-mercury fish. This group also included other big fish—swordfish, for example, and shark.

Why are only large fish a problem? Two reasons. First, big fish eat little fish, and mercury gets concentrated as you move up the food chain. Little fish absorb mercury only from seawater, and therefore typically have low levels of it. Big fish absorb more mercury from the little fish they eat. The bigger the fish, the higher the level of mercury (on average). The second reason is longevity. Bigger fish typically live longer, and the longer they live, the more time they have to accumulate mercury. Sharks can live to be very old, and are therefore chock-full of mercury.

The main concern with eating high-mercury fish is the possible impact on your fetus's developing brain. Mercury is poisonous, and in high doses can cause neurologic damage even in children and adults. For a fetus, even a small dose may matter. In a recent paper, researchers from Harvard went through a number of studies of the impact of mercury on babies. Most of these studies were run in places where people eat *a lot* of fish, so the average levels were much higher than in the United States. The researchers therefore estimated the impact on IQ *per unit* of mercury so that their numbers would be useful to those of us with more limited exposure.[7]

Mercury exposure is measured either through the amount of mercury in Mom's hair or through testing umbilical cord blood. Averaging across a few studies, researchers found that a 1 microgram/gram increase in mercury level led to a decrease of 0.7 IQ points. This effect is fairly small, at least relative to normal mercury levels in the United States. The difference in mercury levels between the average American woman and the most mercury-exposed woman is enough to produce a 3.5-IQ-point difference in their children. Or think about it like this: if you start at the average mercury level and manage to somehow drop your exposure level to zero, this would buy your child, on average, about 1 IQ point.

These effects are small but, hey, every IQ point counts. From this, we'd seem to come to an easy conclusion: do not eat high-mercury fish. I tried hard to avoid these. At work dinners I was typically surreptitiously searching for fish mercury levels on my iPhone under the table. It's not as easy as you'd think. For example: Gulf of Mexico tilefish are terrible, whereas tilefish from the Atlantic are fine. Waiters tend to look at you askance when you ask about the fish origin points. But, on average, you can get a reasonable sense of mercury levels from the FDA, which reports mercury levels for various commercial fish.[8]

But that is not all there is to the story.

Fish—specifically, fish oils—contain very high rates of omega-3 fatty acids. These are *great* for your baby. In particular, they are great for brain development, exactly the thing that mercury is bad for. Published right alongside that study of mercury was a similar study of omega-3 fatty acids, sometimes called DHA. Using evidence from randomized controlled trials of various types of DHA supplementation, the same researchers concluded that increasing your DHA intake by 1 gram per day would increase your child's IQ by, on average, 1.3 points.[9]

How much is 1 gram per day? One serving of salmon has about 1.5 grams of DHA; a serving of tuna has about .5 gram. So this is something like one serving of fish *per day,* probably a lot more than most people eat, and way more than I was managing to eat, especially given the fish restrictions. You *can* get DHA from other sources—most notably, through supplements that come with your prenatal vitamins. But fish are a good source. Several studies have demonstrated that women who consume more fish tend to have children with higher IQs.[10, 11] This means that even with prenatal vitamins and other supplements, more fish is at least correlated with smarter kids.

Making this even more complicated is the fact that fish with a lot of good DHA *are often the same ones* that also have a lot of mercury. Swordfish, for example, is high on the mercury scale and high on the DHA scale.

So what to do?

It turns out that although many fish fall in the high-mercury, high-omega-3 category, not all fish overlap. I ended up with a chart—an "Approval Matrix," if you will—that maps out where various fish fall in the mercury-versus-DHA debate. The fish in the top right quadrant are the best: these are fish that are high in omega-3s but low in mercury, such as herring and sardines (small, oily fish) and salmon. Eating more of these fish can be nothing but good. Three ounces of sardines a day would have a huge impact on your omega-3 intake, but virtually no effect on mercury level.

Other fish—those on the bottom left—are obviously bad. Take something like orange roughy (not a *super* common choice, but not totally unknown): not a lot of omega-3s and a whole load of mercury. Sadly, my favorite choice of canned tuna is in this area, as well.

And then there are those in the middle. The fish on the bottom right—tilefish, swordfish, sushi-grade tuna—are ambiguous. Although they are high in mercury, they also have a lot of omega-3s. You make your kid a little less smart with the mercury, and a little smarter with the omega-3s. They're obviously not as good as the herring and sardines, but they're a lot better than the grouper and the orange roughy. Faced with a choice between canned tuna and sushi tuna, the sushi-grade tuna is, surprisingly, probably a better choice. It's a little higher in mercury, but a lot higher in DHA.

You're typically not forced into eating any particular kind of fish, though, and when you do have a choice, your best option is to stay in the upper-right quadrant. This is true during pregnancy, but also after: the same DHA exposure benefits your baby while you are breast-feeding. You may not be used to eating herring and sardines on a regular basis, but they are worth a shot. My

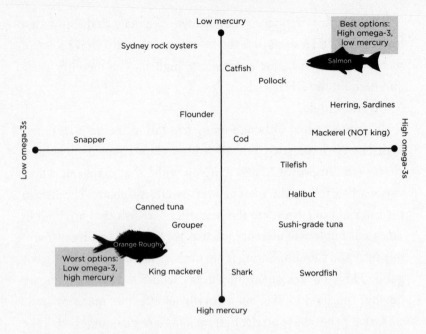

Low mercury

Best options:
High omega-3,
low mercury

Sydney rock oysters

Catfish

Salmon

Pollock

Herring, Sardines

Flounder

Mackerel (NOT king)

Low omega-3s

High omega-3s

Snapper

Cod

Tilefish

Halibut

Canned tuna

Sushi-grade tuna

Grouper

Orange Roughy

Worst options:
Low omega-3,
high mercury

King mackerel

Shark

Swordfish

High mercury

grandmother emigrated from Sweden, and Christmas dinner always features a famous Swedish herring dish: herring, beets, chicken, apples, potatoes, and cream. It takes some getting used to, but think about how smart those Swedish babies must be!

The Bottom Line

- Mercury is bad for your baby. Omega-3 fatty acids are good for your baby. Fish contain both. Your best option is to try to pick fish with a lot of omega-3s and not a lot of mercury.

- The worst thing you can take from the mercury advice is the idea that you should avoid fish. Fish are great! People who eat a lot of fish have smarter kids on average, *even with the greater mercury exposure*. Try to pick smart, and learn to love sardines!

Nausea and My Mother-in-law

Even before I got pregnant, my mother-in-law, Joyce, liked to regale me with her stories of morning sickness. As she tells it, she was deathly ill while pregnant with Jesse, and was saved only by a wonder drug, Bendectin, which at least allowed her to function. Unfortunately, between 1979 (when Jesse was born) and 1985 (when Jesse's sister, Emily, was born), this drug was taken off the market. Joyce was sick nonstop for the entire nine months of her second pregnancy with no relief. Of course she wouldn't have considered taking a drug that had been recalled because of fetal risks, but not being able to eat for the entire pregnancy wasn't so good either. In the end, she gained only eighteen pounds, far below the recommended amount. With the benefit of hindsight, she still wonders: what was so bad about the Bendectin? After all, the first kid turned out fine.

Joyce's level of nausea was unusual, but it is not unheard of. I had at least one friend with a similar experience, and many more who suffered through the first trimester. Nausea is not the only discomfort of pregnancy, but it is probably the most pregnancy-specific. Sure, many women get more headaches while pregnant (lack of caffeine, I suspect). But you've very likely had a headache before, and you know how to treat it.

In contrast, most of us are lucky enough *not* to be throwing up five times a day normally. I know how to deal with the occasional stomach flu by lying in bed and letting Jesse bring me ginger ale, but it's not really an option to rest all day for weeks and weeks, and I suspect Jesse would eventually get tired of waiting on me. Addressing pregnancy-induced nausea is a whole new world, full of drugs and natural remedies that probably never come up in everyday life.

To be clear at the beginning: despite the loss of Joyce's beloved Bendectin, there are drugs that can reduce pregnancy-induced nausea. A popular one is Zofran, which is available by prescription and by all accounts is pretty effective. But even with their discomfort, most women I know are naturally nervous about taking drugs to deal with nausea. Doctors often (not always) reinforce this. Dwyer, the friend with the terrible nausea, was told that she could take Zofran if she "really felt like she needed it." Maybe her doctor didn't intend for this to have a chilling effect, but it did: she came away thinking it was dangerous for her baby, but if she cared only about herself she could take it. Who would be comfortable taking anything at that point?

For many women, an important part of this decision seems to be understanding how their level of nausea compares to the "average" pregnant woman. It's actually not completely clear why this is: for a perfectly rational decision maker, what should matter is how *you* feel about the nausea, not other people's experiences. But in reality, at least the women I know would likely tough it out through an average level of nausea, and think about drug options only if their experiences were unusual.

What is normal? Almost 90 percent of women report some symptoms of nausea and more than half report some vomiting as well.[1] This tends to peak at around 8 or 9 weeks of pregnancy and fall off after that. The graph below gives you a sense of how many women report being sick by week of pregnancy.[2] Almost 50 percent of the women in this study reported vomiting at some point in weeks 5 to 8 of pregnancy, but it was less than 15 to 20 percent by 17 weeks.

Although it's probably reassuring to know that for most women the nausea eventually goes away, this graph does suggest that the resolution isn't immediate when you enter the second trimester. If you've been very sick for the first few weeks, you shouldn't expect to feel great as soon as you hit week 13 or 14, although things should be gradually improving at that point.

Some amount of nausea is normal. But if you are so sick you can't keep anything down and aren't able to function at all, you might start to wonder whether this is *really* normal. To answer this, we can get a little more detailed. In one study of 2,500

Share of Women Reporting Vomiting, by Pregnancy Week

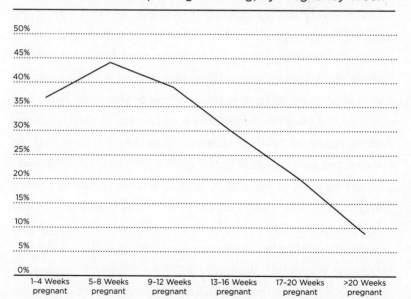

women, at the worst point in her pregnancy, the average person was throwing up at least once a day, and about 13 percent of them were throwing up at least 3 times a day.[3] And as for the name "morning" sickness, it's a serious misnomer: in another study with detailed data of the timing of nausea over the course of the day, more than 80 percent of the women reported that they felt sick all day, not just in the morning.[4] But the number of days of actual vomiting for women in these studies was actually small: only an average of 6 bad days over the course of the pregnancy.

What does this mean, putting it all together? The average pregnant woman starts to feel bad at around 6 weeks (that's two weeks after her missed period). She starts feeling better at around 13 or 14 weeks, a couple of weeks into the second trimester. During this time, she may or may not throw up at all. If she does, it will typically be concentrated in just a few days (although those days might be quite bad). If you are throwing up every day for a month, that is unusual: in these studies, only about 5 percent of women report nausea that severe.[5]

Very severe nausea has another name: *hyperemesis gravidarum*. This is typically defined as frequent vomiting (a rule of thumb is more than 3 times a day) accompanied by other complications (dehydration, weight loss, low potassium).[6] Nausea this severe is actually quite dangerous for both Mom and baby, and can lead to low birth weight and higher rates of preterm birth. Almost 1 percent of all pregnant women are sick enough to be hospitalized for this (usually the main problem is dehydration).[7] This can be scary in addition to uncomfortable and many women worry that they will not be able to eat enough to nourish their baby. Good news here: if you eventually gain an appropriate amount of weight after the nausea resolves, there do not seem to be adverse effects on baby size.

If you have read this and discovered you're above average in terms of nausea, and are now cursing your body for failing you, hold off a minute. As unpleasant as it is, nausea is a sign of a healthy pregnancy. Miscarriage rates are much lower for women who are nauseated than for those who are not. In early pregnancy the differences can be quite large: one study showed that the overall risk of first-trimester miscarriage was 30 percent for women without nausea, versus just 8 percent for those who were nauseated.[8]

Knowing this, the sicker I felt in the morning during my first trimester, the happier Jesse was. There is nothing quite like waking up, feeling terrible, and having your spouse tell you how excited he is that you feel bad. I don't think I've ever seen him quite as happy as the one day I actually threw up.

It may be reassuring to know that sickness is a sign of a healthy pregnancy, but for actually feeling better, you'll need to think about some kind of treatment. And the truth is that even if your nausea is not so severe that you're in hospitalization territory, debilitating nausea can be more than just inconvenient. Hydration and nourishment is important for your pregnancy; if you can't keep anything down, it could pose a problem. Just sitting around and suffering through it is certainly not great for you, and it may not be great for the baby either.

Usually the first step is the simple stuff you are doing anyway: eat only what you can tolerate and don't eat much at once, have some crackers before you get out of bed, and so on. For a while, Jane's husband, Dave, spent much of his time trying to find food that she could stomach. Chef Boyardee played a major role.

If this doesn't work, you are going to want to look for something a bit more concrete. The general distrust of prescription drugs during pregnancy has led many women to look first for some holistic or natural remedy for nausea. Options include things like ginger or vitamins, which are often used to treat normal nonpregnancy nausea, as well as acupuncture and acupressure.

As it turns out, evidence on the effectiveness of these interventions is fairly limited and not terribly encouraging.

A recent review of randomized studies found no support for either acupressure or acupuncture in reducing nausea. A couple of small studies did show some benefit from ginger (typically prepared in a tea), but the studies are of somewhat limited quality. One thing that does seem to work is vitamin B6: randomized trials suggest a reduction in nausea from relatively high doses. B6 is safe; it's actually found in your prenatal vitamins, although at doses lower than you'd need to combat sickness. In the trials, it seemed to be most effective against mild nausea and had no impact on actual vomiting.[9]

If you are sick enough to be looking for something a bit stronger than a can of ginger ale, you'll want to look into the drug options. Drugs for nausea in pregnancy have a long and troubled history. In the late 1950s many women were prescribed thalidomide to address pregnancy nausea. It's not even clear if this worked as a treatment for nausea, but it did cause serious birth defects. Estimates suggest it affected perhaps ten thousand births before being taken off the market in the early 1960s.[10]

Later, in the 1970s and 1980s, women (like Jesse's mom) were often prescribed Bendectin. Joyce's positive experience was not unusual. Randomized controlled trials of the drug show positive effects on nausea and vomiting, improved well-being, and some (not quite significant) impacts on lost time in employment. At the end of at least one trial, 50 percent of the women wanted to keep using the drug, versus 30 percent of the women taking a placebo, suggesting the drug was more effective than a sugar pill.[11]

In 1983, Bendectin was taken off the market in the United States. To understand why, we need to understand that some babies are born with birth defects even if their mothers take no drugs during pregnancy and do everything perfectly. There is just some baseline risk of birth defects in the population. Bendectin was prescribed to many, many women. And some of their babies had birth defects. Perhaps because of the thalidomide experience in the 1950s, some women who took Bendectin and had babies with birth defects found their way to lawyers. In the early 1980s, those lawyers brought a suit against the makers of Bendectin, claiming that the drug caused the birth defects. The makers of the drug, facing millions of dollars in legal fees even if they ultimately won the suit, pulled the drug from the market. This actually gives us another source of information on the effectiveness of the drug, and supports it. When it was pulled from the market, hospitalizations for severe nausea doubled.[12]

The FDA was naturally worried. They had approved the drug in the first place; had they made a mistake? As it turns out, no. In response to the lawsuit, several papers collated the studies on Bendectin. A 1994 review included twenty-seven studies comparing women who did and did not take Bendectin.[13] They found that women who had exposure to Bendectin in the first trimester had children with slightly *fewer* birth defects, and statistically, they couldn't prove that there was any difference between the two groups.

In light of this extremely reassuring evidence, the drug retained its FDA approval in the United States. However, the threat of lawsuits loomed, and Bendectin never came back on the market in the United States.

This is particularly ridiculous because the drug is actually just a combination of two over the counter items—vitamin B6 and Unisom—both of which are considered safe in pregnancy. In the absence of a single pill solution, doctors and women have made use of this "roll-your-own" Bendectin option for years.

If this doesn't work, there are a number of stronger prescription drugs for nausea. Options include promethazine and Zofran (the two most common) and a few others (such as metoclopramide and compazine). In general, evidence from studies of animals and small-scale studies in people suggest that these drugs are safe and at least somewhat effective.[14] Steroids are also sometimes used, although these seem to increase the risk of cleft lip and palate if they are given in the first trimester, so they tend to be used only if there is no improvement with the other medications.[15]

I know a lot of women who were really pretty sick in their first trimester. Yet I know only one who actually took any prescription drugs. At first, I attributed this problem to reluctance from doctors to prescribe medication. That idea really riled up some of my OB friends. My medical editor, Emily, was surprised: "I certainly don't hesitate to prescribe medications for nausea—better to get out ahead so they don't get *really* sick." And as I talked to more women, and to more doctors, it dawned on me: maybe the holdup in this case was *us*.

At one point I spoke with a woman on an airplane who had a child about Penelope's age. She reported to me that during her first trimester she threw up 10 to 15 times a day for 12 weeks. I asked why she didn't try any medications. She told me she had never even asked her doctor about them, and she just wasn't comfortable with the idea of medication during pregnancy.

Sure, it's possible that your doctor will be reluctant to prescribe you medication, or may first suggest you try eating smaller meals. But it increasingly seems to me that it's the women who are reluctant to ask, who think they should suffer in silence. That's not always a great idea: serious dehydration and weight loss during pregnancy can lead to complications. Why risk it when there are good, safe treatment options?

The Bottom Line

- Some nausea is normal and is probably a good sign about pregnancy.

- Vomiting every day for weeks is more than the average person experiences.

- Treatment (in order): (1) small meals, (2) vitamin B6 + ginger ale, (3) Vitamin B6 + Unisom (or Diclegis, with a prescription), (4) Zofran.

. . .

Prenatal Screening and Testing

There is one major medical decision to be made in the first trimester of pregnancy: prenatal screening. I was prepared for this one. Before getting pregnant I'd been doing research on genetic testing; I'd been immersed in the academic literature on this for months. Even though my research wasn't specifically about *prenatal* testing, I couldn't help but read a few papers on it (for work purposes, of course!).

Jesse and I started talking about the right thing to do almost as soon as we found out I was pregnant. The first weekend after that conference we were on a vacation with my family and I spent a reasonable part of the weekend on my computer, trying to get to the bottom of this issue.

More than anything else in pregnancy, making the right decision about this depends on having the right decision framework—about correctly weighing the pluses and minuses of different choices. Of course, this is really what economics is designed for.

Perhaps most important, making this decision depends on thinking about these pluses and minuses *for you, personally*. I'd argue that no two people will think about this decision quite the same way. Which is why even having a "standard" recommendation here makes so little sense to me—even less than it does elsewhere.

But a little background first.

The goal of all prenatal screening and testing is the same: to learn whether your baby has a chromosomal abnormality. Human DNA has twenty-three pairs of chromosomes. The vast majority of chromosomal problems are caused by having three copies of a chromosome rather than the normal amount of just two. For most of the chromosomes, a fetus with three copies will not survive—you'll have an early miscarriage, or you'll never know you were pregnant at all.

In a few cases, however, survival is possible or likely. By far, the most common of these is Down syndrome, which is caused by having three copies of chromosome 21. Down syndrome is characterized by some degree of mental retardation and distinctive facial features, among other things. The two other common ones are Edwards syndrome (three copies of chromosome 18) and Patau syndrome (three copies of chromosome 13). These are more severe than Down syndrome; babies born with these conditions rarely survive their first year.

The risk to your baby of any of these conditions depends on your age. I've included a quick reference table, along with some comparisons to probabilities you might be more familiar with.[1]

I was 31 when Penelope was born. This put my risk around 1 in 700. This means that of 700 women my age who get pregnant, on average 1 of them will carry a baby with Down syndrome. By the time my son, Finn, was born I was thirty-five. That put my risk up to 1 in 374.

Prior to the advent of prenatal testing, women wouldn't learn about whether their child had one of these conditions until they were born. By the time my mother was pregnant with me and my brothers, some women were offered a test for these conditions (called an amniocentesis) in their second trimester. This test

Risk of Down Syndrome by Age . . .

Age	Chance of Down Syndrome
20–24	1 in 1488
25–29	1 in 1118
30–34	1 in 746
35	1 in 374
36	1 in 289
37	1 in 224
38	1 in 173
39	1 in 136
40	1 in 106
41	1 in 82
42	1 in 63
43	1 in 49
44	1 in 38
45	1 in 30

. . . and Some Comparisons

Car accident in next year: 1 in 50

Audited next year: 1 in 200

Injury with fireworks: 1 in 19,000

Winning Powerball: 1 in 80 million

accurately detects Down syndrome and the other chromosomal abnormalities, but carries a small risk of miscarriage. Because of the relationship between these problems and maternal age, it was common to offer this test only to women over 35.

The amniocentesis is still around. It's been joined by another procedure called *chorionic villus sampling* (CVS for short), which can be done earlier in the pregnancy but also carries some risk of miscarriage. In addition, in the last twenty years doctors have made enormous progress on prenatal *screening*. The older version of this screening—which was available when I had Penelope and is still in use—uses information from an ultrasound and a blood test along with your age. The newer version—which came around by the time I had Finn—uses a blood test alone to sequence fetal DNA.

The advantage to either screening option is that it carries no miscarriage risk. The disadvantage is that it cannot tell you *for sure* whether your baby is affected. No matter the results, there will still be some (perhaps very small) probability that your baby has a chromosomal problem that you'll learn about at birth.

As I outlined for Jesse, we had three options:

Option 1: Do nothing. We could avoid any testing altogether. The risk of a chromosomal problem would be determined only by my age, and we would learn the truth when the baby arrived.

Option 2: Start with the prenatal screening. The doctor could do the screening tests, and, at the end, they'd tell us some new risk (could be higher or lower than the baseline). Then, depending on the results, we could choose to do invasive testing.

Option 3: Skip right to the invasive testing (either an amnio-centesis or a CVS test). This would mean a procedure with some risk, but it would tell us for sure whether our baby had a normal set of chromosomes.

For us, option 1 was out. As will presumably come as no surprise given the themes of this book, we tend to want more information rather than less. Because the noninvasive testing (option 2) carries no risk to the baby, we knew we would at least do that. Of course, not everyone feels this way. I've had more than one person tell me that they knew they would continue the pregnancy no matter what, and they didn't want to risk a "bad" test result that would make them worry more than necessary. A thoughtful view, if not ours.

We were then left with option 2 versus option 3. I explained to

Jesse a bit how the tests worked. If we went with the noninvasive option, at the end of the testing we'd know more, but still have some remaining risk. If we went with the invasive testing, we'd know for sure, but there was some risk.

"Thanks, this is helpful," Jesse wrote (we were doing this over e-mail; you would be surprised how much better that is for complicated analyses). "But I don't have enough information. If the noninvasive testing goes well, what will the remaining risk be? And how risky is the CVS or amniocentesis (and, for that matter, which of those would we want to do?). —Jesse."

He was right, of course (rare, but it does occasionally happen). In order to make this decision we needed to know those numbers. Alone, they were *still* not going to be enough information, because we'd have to consider our personal feelings about having a miscarriage or a baby with a disability. But we couldn't even start that discussion without knowing the data.

I got to work.

At my 10-week prenatal visit, I asked my doctor. She had recommended the screening test (the noninvasive option), so I asked a simple form of my question. If that test went well, what would my risk be? I was told it would be "very low."

"How low?" I asked. "One in a thousand? One in ten thousand? One in thirty thousand?"

"Yes," was the response, "something like that."

I am willing to accept that I'm perhaps a little more neurotic about exact numbers than most people, but this seemed extremely vague: 1 in 1,000 and 1 in 30,000 are quite different. To put it in perspective, 1 in 1,000 pregnant women have their babies delivered by a midwife rather than a doctor; it is unusual, sure, but I would be willing to bet you know people in this group. In contrast, 1 in 30,000 is the risk of going to the ER this year for an injury involving a blanket (no, I am not making this up).[2] I would be willing to bet you do not know anyone this has happened to.

These tests were run at an office different from my normal doctor; the office was staffed with a genetic counselor. Surely that person would be better at answering these questions. Not really. After a good test result, the ultimate conclusion was that I had the risk of a 20-year-old. That sounds great, but what does it mean? A 20-year-old who also had a good test result? A 20-year-old with no test? This was accompanied by a little bar graph that showed how my actual age of 31 was much higher than my "genetic age" of 20. Needless to say, this didn't really clear it up. I still have no idea what was meant by "genetic age."

My doctor wasn't much better on the risk of miscarriage from the invasive-testing options. I got a concrete number (a risk of miscarriage of about 1 in 200 for amniocentesis), but it turned out to be the same number that my mother was told back in 1985. It was hard for me to believe that things hadn't improved.

I realized that if I wanted an answer to either of these questions I'd have to do some digging on my own. I started out by trying to figure out exactly how these screening tests worked and then moved on to figuring out the risks from the invasive testing.

In the end, this is one of the few parts of pregnancy I had to research twice—first with Penelope and then with Finn. The fundamental decision process didn't change between pregnancies, but the technology did. By the time I was expecting Finn, a new blood test had dramatically improved the accuracy of the noninvasive screening options. Jesse and I once again discussed these (by now we had moved from e-mail to a family task-management system) and, once again, found that we needed the data. There was still no "correct" answer and still no answer at all without the numbers.

Noninvasive Prenatal Screening

Conceptually, prenatal screening is simple. The goal is to find some characteristic of the fetus or some marker in the maternal blood that is more common for babies who have Down syndrome or another chromosomal abnormality. You can then use this characteristic to provide more information to parents about the chance that their baby is affected.

It may be easier to understand the basic idea with a nonpregnancy-related example. Consider the much less emotionally fraught process of shopping for fruit. At the store you're faced with a selection of cantaloupes, and you want to make sure the one you choose is ripe. In order to know *for sure* whether a particular one is ripe you'd have to cut into it and taste it. This, of course, isn't possible to do before you buy.

What you likely do instead is try to figure out whether the fruit is ripe by looking at things you can see on the outside. What color is it? How does it smell? People have all sorts of tricks for doing this. Someone once told me you can figure this out based on whether the fruit is especially heavy. Whatever your personal system is, it's all the same theory. Take the color. On average, melons that have some green rind are less likely to be ripe. If you see a melon with no green rind, therefore, you think it's more likely to be ripe. A statistician would say that you are trying to *infer the truth* (whether or not it is ripe) *based on a signal* (in this case, whether or not the rind is green).

Using these techniques, you pick the cantaloupe you think is most likely to be ripe and you buy it. But you know that no matter how good your tricks are, there is still some risk. There is some chance that when you get home and cut into the melon, you will find it is not ripe. Some of the cantaloupes that look ready are not. On the flip side, there are some cantaloupes in the bin that get left behind because they don't look ripe—they are green, or they don't smell much—and yet they actually *are* ripe. These are two different kinds of "mistakes." In the first case, you think everything is fine, but it is not. In the second, you think there is a problem, but there isn't.

This example may seem completely unrelated—and, in terms of emotional valence and importance, it no doubt is!—but, in terms of the statistics, this is very similar to how the first trimester screening works. Doctors want to identify babies who are healthy (the ripe melons in the example above). They have found some features that are more common among healthy babies or healthy pregnancies (in the example, no green on the cantaloupe rind). If they see these signs, this makes it more likely that the baby is healthy.

This basic analysis description applies to either screening test. The exact way they work (and their accuracy), however, differs a bit between the current state-of-the-art, cell-free fetal DNA screening and the older ultrasound and blood test screenings.

Cell Fee Fetal DNA

It has been known for decades that some fetal cells circulate in the maternal blood stream during pregnancy. If it were possible to isolate those cells—to separate them from Mom's—this would enable fetal genetic sequencing without any invasive testing. The key to the accuracy of amniocentesis or CVS testing is that these procedures access and test actual fetal cells. If that were possible without invasive testing, it would deliver the best of both worlds.

Progress in this area was, however, impeded by the fact that the concentration of fetal cells in maternal blood is extremely low. This made it difficult or impossible to get enough blood to isolate a sufficient concentration of fetal cells.

In the late 1990s, however, researchers discovered that cell-free fetal DNA—fetal DNA that exists outside of cells—mixes at much higher concentrations with maternal cell-free DNA. When cell-free DNA is isolated in maternal plasma, 10 to 20 percent of it is fetal in origin.[3] This higher concentration has made it possible to improve prenatal screening.

In principle, if it were possible to simply separate the maternal and fetal DNA, it would be possible to sequence the full fetal DNA using this procedure. The technology is still not quite there on that—although it is improving. Instead, this procedure works by looking for things in the cell-free DNA that wouldn't be there if it were just the mom.

The simplest way to illustrate this is with gender. Women have two X chromosomes, men have one X and one Y. Imagine you look in Mom's cell-free DNA and you find a bunch of Y chromosomes. Since you can be sure they are not from her, they must be from the baby, and the baby must, therefore, be a boy. Conversely, if you do not see any Y chromosomes, this increases the confidence the baby is a girl.

This procedure can be used in a similar way to test for chromosomal abnormalities. Take Down syndrome as an example. A fetus with Down syndrome has three, rather than two, copies of chromosome 21 but two copies of all of the other chromosomes. Assuming the mother does not have any chromosomal abnormalities, she has two copies of all chromosomes, including chromosome 21. This means if you look at a mix of fetal and maternal DNA together, if the baby has Down syndrome, the DNA will have relatively more copies of chromosome 21 than of the other chromosomes.

To simplify this somewhat, the way the technology works is to look for these types of imbalances and, if the imbalance is striking enough, flag the test result as possibly indicating a chromosomal problem.

In the end, you will be told the test result is either positive, meaning there is some evidence of a problem and further screening is recommended, or negative, meaning that the chromosomes look balanced and no further screening is recommended.

Just like with the fruit, these procedures cannot tell you *for sure* whether or not the baby has Down syndrome. Sometimes the imbalance in the chromosome counts isn't striking enough to flag as a positive test, even when the baby does have a chromosomal abnormality. This is what is called a *false negative*. And on the other side, sometimes the chromosome looks imbalanced but the baby is fine. This is what is called a *false positive*.

Once I understood the underlying principles here, I took a step back and thought about the process. If we went ahead with the screening, at the end of the day the result would be a recommendation from my doctor. If my tests went well, she would recommend I do nothing else. If they didn't go well, she would recommend more testing, either a CVS or amniocentesis. The key question for me was how much information is really provided by a "positive" versus a "negative" result.

This crystallized for me what I needed to know. First, I needed to know how accurate these tests were at detecting chromosomal problems. If my final risk was above the cutoff and they told me "Everything is great, do nothing!" how confident could I be? What percent of babies with chromosomal problems are missed by this test?

Second, I need to know how likely it was that there would be a false positive—that is, that the doctor would say that there was more testing necessary when, in fact, the baby was fine. My reasoning was that if this was very common, that would favor skipping right to the CVS or amniocentesis. If I was probably going to do that anyway, why should I go through the anxiety of being told I had a "bad" screening result, then worry for weeks before getting a final answer?

The answer to my first question is that about 99 percent of trisomies are detected with this procedure. The largest available study of this was run in China and published in 2015.[4] This study covered almost 147,000 women who underwent this testing. There were 726 cases of Down syndrome among their children, of which the test detected 720, or about 99.1%. A similar detection rate is found in earlier studies that focused on high-risk women,[5] although this large study is especially nice because it shows similar detection rates in a low-risk population.

This large study also answered my second question on the false positive rate. In this case, 781 women were told they had a positive screen for Down syndrome, and 720 of these were confirmed by later diagnosis. This means that 61 women were given a false positive. This can be converted to a false positive rate that measures the share of women with a healthy baby who are told that they have a positive screen; in this population, which is huge, the share is 0.05 percent, or about 5 women out of 10,000. In other words, of 10,000 women tested, 5 of them will be told their fetus has screened positive for a chromosomal problem, but, in fact, the fetus is chromosomally normal.

These data gave me the relevant numbers, but they didn't entirely answer Jesse's question. What he really wanted at the end of the day was a risk: If the test result was good, what was the remaining chance of a chromosomal problem? To answer this, it is necessary to combine these figures with the baseline risk by age. The table below shows these calculations. The first column of numbers is the estimate of Down syndrome risk if you have a negative test result. The second is the risk if you have a positive test result.

For me, there are really two striking things to take away from this table. First, the detection rates from this test are excellent. With a negative test result, the remaining risk—while not zero—is

Age	Chance of Down syndrome with negative test result	Chance of Down syndrome with positive test result
20–24	1 in 179,830	1 in 1.8
25–29	1 in 135,085	1 in 1.6
30–34	1 in 90,097	1 in 1.4
35	1 in 45,109	1 in 1.2
36	1 in 34,830	1 in 1.15
37	1 in 26,969	1 in 1.12
38	1 in 20,801	1 in 1.09
39	1 in 16,327	1 in 1.07
40	1 in 12,699	1 in 1.06
41	1 in 9,796	1 in 1.04
42	1 in 7,498	1 in 1.03
43	1 in 5,805	1 in 1.03
44	1 in 4,475	1 in 1.02
45	1 in 3,508	1 in 1.01

very small. Second—and this is very important to keep in mind—the false positive rates mean that even if you do have a positive test result, for most age groups the actual chance of having a baby with Down syndrome is still not 100 percent. For the youngest age group—women in their early twenties—the chance of Down syndrome with a positive test result is still only about 50 percent. For older women a positive test result is extremely likely to indicate a problem, with a risk of about 98 percent.

This table was the answer to at least part of what I needed to know when pregnant with Finn. I was 35 at his delivery. With a good result on this screening test, the remaining risk of a chromosomal problem was about 1 in about 45,000. With a bad result on the test, although it was not certain, the chance that he was affected was over 80 percent.

Ultrasound + Blood Test, First Trimester Screen

The cell-free fetal DNA technology described above has become increasingly common, but for many women it will still not be covered by insurance. In my case, it was covered only because by the time I got around to having Finn I was over 35 and, therefore, considered "high risk." If this is not accessible to you, you are likely to be offered an older technology that involves an ultrasound and a blood test for hormone levels.

The most useful measurement taken in these tests is an ultrasound measure of the amount of fluid behind the baby's neck (called the *nuchal translucency*, or *NT*). Fetuses who have Down syndrome are much more likely to have a lot of fluid behind the neck. Doctors also measure two hormones in Mom's blood (PAPP-A and hCG). Women who are carrying fetuses with Down syndrome also tend to have different hormone levels from those whose babies have normal chromosomes. By comparing your measurements and hormone levels to those of fetuses with and without Down syndrome, your doctor can learn about your baby's health.

The results of this test have the same basic structure as the results from the cell-free tests. You will either screen positive or negative, with the former indicating further testing is needed and the latter indicating that further testing is not suggested. The big difference between this and the newer technology is in the accuracy.

This test detect about 90 percent of cases of Down syndrome, versus 99 percent for the newer tests.[6, 7] The false positive rate is also much higher—at about 6.3 percent (versus 0.05 percent). For every 100 women who have this test, 6 of them will be told they have screened positive and then subsequently learn their infants are healthy. This is in contrast to 5 in 10,000 for the newer test. This means the overall performance of the tests is worse.

It is also worth noting that the performance of this test differs significantly by age. Detection rates are much lower for younger women (only about 85 percent for women in their late twenties), and false positive rates are extremely high for older women (close to 50 percent for women in their early forties).*

If you do go with this option rather than the newer testing, some doctors will offer further screening in the second trimester, around 15 to 18 weeks of pregnancy. At this stage more blood is drawn from Mom, and it is tested for four additional hormones: alpha-fetoprotein, hCG, unconjugated estriol, and inhibin A. Doctors use these exactly the same way they use the data from the first trimester; in fact, they usually combine the two sets of results. Using everything together, doctors can detect an even larger percentage of babies with Down syndrome—as many as 97 percent of cases.[8]

Other Conditions

Most of the discussion of prenatal screening focuses on Down syndrome, probably because it is the most common chromosomal abnormality. However, this same screening procedure is also effective at detecting trisomy 18 and trisomy 13 (Edwards and Patau syndromes, respectively). These conditions are much rarer—trisomy 18 occurs in about 1 out of 5,000 live births, and trisomy 13 in 1 out of 10,000—and both are typically fatal within the

---

* A technical note: this happens because your final risk depends, in part, on your age. For someone who is 45, her baseline risk of a baby with Down syndrome is about 1 in 30. Even if her test results look great, there is still some fairly high risk that her baby is affected, just because the baseline rate is so high. This means that most women who are 45 and undergo this screening are told they are positive—it's just mechanical. Only 45-year-old women with really fantastic, amazing test results are told they are negative; this means that nearly all of them do, in fact, have healthy babies. But on the other hand, many 45-year-old women with good test results are told they are positive just because of the baseline risk, so the false positive rate is high. The converse is true for a younger person. Because the baseline level of risk is fairly low, only if her test results are quite bad is she told to do more screening. But this means that the detection rate is lower because some women with pretty bad test results are still told they are fine.

first year of life. The risk of these conditions also varies by age. The risk of either condition under age 25 is around 1 in 5,500, and it is as high as 1 in 162 for women age 45.

The screening test for these diseases works just like described above, only better: detection rates are very good (much better than for Down syndrome), and false positives are rare. The cell-free procedures detect these nearly perfectly, and even the older screening technologies are quite good. In a 2002 paper, two authors from the United Kingdom reported that the ultrasound and blood test option can detect 95 percent of cases, with a 0.3 percent false positive rate.[9] Because the risks are low to begin with and the screening procedure is so good, after a good screen the remaining risk of either condition is very, very small.

The Bottom Line: Part 1

- Cell-free fetal DNA testing (MaterniT21, Harmony, and others) are very accurate and can detect about 99 percent of Down syndrome cases.

- False positives are rare, but they do happen.

- If these tests are not available, first-trimester screening with ultrasound and blood tests can detect about 90 percent of Down syndrome cases but with higher false positive rates.

Invasive Prenatal Testing: CVS and Amniocentesis

I spent a tremendous amount of time in both pregnancies on this noninvasive stuff, and I was still only half done with Jesse's questions. The other testing option (which I could do in addition to *or* instead of the screening) was an invasive prenatal test, either a CVS test or an amniocentesis. Both of these tests would allow my doctor (or, more accurately, some lab) to actually sequence fetal DNA and would tell us for sure if the chromosomes looked normal. But both involved a needle going into the uterus, and therefore both carried some small risk of miscarriage. But I still didn't know how small. And I didn't know that much about how the two tests compared.

The procedures involve the same basic method: the doctor goes into the uterus with a needle and takes a sample of the baby's cells. There are two differences: where those cells come from and at what stage of pregnancy the procedure is performed.

Inside the uterus, the baby is surrounded by the fluid-filled amniotic sac; this fluid is full of the baby's cells. For an amniocentesis, the doctor inserts a long, (very) thin needle through your belly into the uterus and into the amniotic sac (they use a local anesthetic to numb you). They take out some of the amniotic fluid, separate out the cells that belong to you, and look directly at the baby's chromosomes. This procedure is typically performed between 16 and 20 weeks of pregnancy (doing it much earlier appears to increase the risk of club foot, so is generally avoided).[10]

Amniocentesis has been around for decades. CVS is newer—it was introduced in the early 1980s—but its use has grown since then. In a CVS test, the cells are taken from the placenta. Again, the doctor goes in with a needle, either through the abdomen or through the cervix, and grabs a few placenta cells. As with amniocentesis, they separate out any cells that belong to Mom and, again, look at the baby's chromosomes. CVS is performed much earlier in the pregnancy, typically between 10 and 12 weeks, before the end of the first trimester.

In both cases the risks to the pregnant woman herself are vanishingly small, and recovery typically takes only a day or two.

Once the cells have been taken, doctors can use a "fast" procedure (called *fluorescence in situ hybridization*, or FISH) to test for the most common problems (trisomy 13 and 18, and Down syndrome) and to learn the sex of the baby. These results are available within a couple of days after the test. A more complete (and more accurate) procedure takes one to two weeks, at which point you can see the full set of baby chromosomes. This is very cool (baby's first genetic sequence!) but it contains little information beyond what they can tell you after a few days, because having extra copies of chromosomes *other than* 13, 18, or 21 is extremely rare.

These tests are accurate. Either one will tell you with an extremely high degree of confidence whether or not your baby is healthy. False negatives or false positives are vanishingly rare.

This accuracy is, of course, the big plus of these tests relative to the screening. On the negative side is the possibility that the tests could cause a miscarriage. In principle, sticking needles into the uterus could certainly carry some danger. You'll often see pretty high risks cited for these procedures (by your doctor or by the popular pregnancy books). Common numbers are a 1 in 100 risk of miscarriage from CVS, and 1 in 200 from amniocentesis.

When I sat down to research this the most striking fact was that the risks from either of these procedures are much lower than 1 in 100 or 1 in 200. They are so low that it's hard even to put a figure on it, but my best estimate was about 1 in 800.

You may be thinking: Where did this 1 in 200 number come from, if not from evidence? And why does anyone still think that amniocentesis is less risky if it is so obvious that it is not?

The answer to the first question is, basically, low-quality historical data. The 1 in 200 figure is based on a study from the 1970s that considered about 1,000 women who underwent amniocentesis and 1,000 matched controls.[11] In the amniocentesis group, 3.5 percent of the women had a miscarriage. In the control group, it was 3.2 percent. *This difference was not statistically significant and disappeared completely when corrected for maternal age.* In lay terms, this means that the study actually didn't show *any* increased risk of miscarriage from amniocentesis. And yet, the 1 in 200 number was born.

This was bolstered by a study in the 1980s that did a better job in various ways and suggested a similar risk. But even this study is hard to learn from, in large part because it is old.[12]

Old studies are not always useless. Some things do not change much over a period of thirty years. But some things do, and the technology for doing these tests is definitely in that category. The biggest changes have to do with the use of ultrasound during these procedures.

The most significant risk of these tests is that you accidentally hit the fetus with the needle; a related risk is the needle going through the placenta, which can also cause problems. It used to be that doctors would do an ultrasound before starting and then make a guess about the best way to go in. If the baby moved, they might have guessed wrong. Today, doctors typically watch what they are doing the entire time on the ultrasound. This means there is basically no risk of either hitting the baby or going through the placenta. Adding to those improvements, the quality of ultrasound technology has dramatically increased in the last decades. The better picture makes it easier for the doctor to see what she is doing and lowers the risks.

Fortunately, there are some newer studies of amniocentesis. And, not surprisingly, they show much lower risks. One good one is the FASTER trial.[13] This was a study originally designed to evaluate the noninvasive screening options, but some women in the study chose to undergo invasive screening as well.

Researchers compared the miscarriage rates for women in this study who underwent an amniocentesis to those who were also in the study but chose not to have this procedure. The chance of

pregnancy loss before 24 weeks was 0.94 percent in the control
(no amniocentesis) group and 1.0 percent in the treatment (amniocentesis) group. This difference is very small—it would suggest a
procedure-related risk of 1 in 1,600—and wasn't significant, meaning we can't conclude that there is *any* additional risk to the baby.

Two other recent studies used a similar design, comparing
women who had an amniocentesis to similar women who did not,
and found the same results. Neither study showed a difference in
miscarriage rates between the amniocentesis and no-amniocente-
sis groups. Again, we can't reject the claim that there is *no* increase
in risk from the procedure. If we take the magnitude of their
estimates seriously, they suggest a procedure-related risk around
1 in 800.[14]

The case of CVS is a bit more complicated. This procedure has
been around for much less time, and it is also a slightly more
complex procedure to perform. This means there is a substantial
learning component, and, over time, the risks from the procedure
have gone down as it has gotten more common.

We can see this directly in one interesting study that focuses on
comparing these two procedures over a twenty year period (from
1983–2003) in one hospital in California.[15] It becomes clear how
much the CVS technology has advanced. In the earliest period of
the study, in the mid-1980s, they estimate the risks from CVS to
be about twenty times higher than amniocentesis! By the 1998–
2003 period, however, they had exactly the same level of risk,
adjusting for Mom's characteristics and the timing of the test.

The current edition of the most popular obstetrics textbook
used in medical schools reviews a number of papers comparing
CVS to amniocentesis and concludes that the risks are the same
in the two cases.[16] This would put the risk of miscarriage from
CVS also around 1 in 800. This low risk would be consistent with
the one well-designed study I found that compared CVS to no
testing and found no statistically significant difference in miscar-

riage rates (in fact, the subsequent miscarriage rate was lower for the group with CVS).[17]

When I was expecting Penelope I was confident that the CVS test would dominate the amniocentesis if we decided to do invasive testing (which we didn't; more on this below). By the time we got around to Finn, I expected this to be even more true as time passed and the CVS technology was more used. As it turned out, this was not the case; I hadn't banked on the role of the improved noninvasive testing.

The main value of CVS is the accurate early test results. The ultrasound-based noninvasive screen is really not that useful for older women, who have a very high rate of false positives, so for women in this group the CVS often dominates. But with the advent of the cell-free fetal DNA testing, chromosomal problems are detected with a high rate of accuracy even for these older women. Many, many people switched from CVS testing to this cell-free screen instead.

Rates of CVS use have dramatically decreased. When I was expecting Finn I asked the genetic counselor about how common this procedure was. She told me that prior to the cell-free testing they were doing close to one test per day, and they were now down to only about one or two a month.

The data I found on CVS clearly indicated that risks had gone down as the procedure became more common, but, by the same token, it seems likely that risks will go up (at least a bit) as the procedure becomes less common. This doesn't mean the CVS test has a risk of 1 in 100—there is no basis for this number anyway—but it did give me more pause.

It is worth saying that although amniocentesis is also now a less used genetic screening, it is used for a lot of other things during pregnancy (testing for lung development close to term, for example) and is a much more straightforward procedure, so there is much less reason to expect a change in the risks.

The Bottom Line: Part 2

- Miscarriage rates from both amniocentesis and CVS are small.

- A reasonable estimate of procedure-related miscarriage risk from amniocentesis is about 1 in 800, although most studies are not large enough to allow us to reject the claim that there is no increased risk from this procedure.

- Most data suggest miscarriage risks from CVS and amniocentesis are indistinguishable, but because CVS has become less common over time, it is important to look for a provider who still does many of these.

Decision Time

Armed with all the data we needed, Jesse and I set about actually making this decision. We did this first with Penelope and then, four years later, with Finn. Between the births of the two kids I had passed the magic number of 35 and was of "advanced maternal age," which meant, interestingly, that the recommended course of action had also changed.

Historically, genetic testing recommendations depended only on age. Women over 35 were offered invasive screening and those under 35 were not. This is based very loosely on comparing probabilities. A woman at age 35 has about a 1 in 200 risk of conceiving a baby with any chromosomal problem. The (historical) estimate of the risk of miscarriage from an amniocentesis was 1 in 200. So someone decided the right way to make this decision was to compare probabilities. Over 35, the risk of a chromosomal problem is higher than the risk of miscarriage, so you should test. Under 35, the miscarriage risk is higher, so you should not.

From a decision perspective—heck, from a basic logic perspective—this is insane. One reason, of course, is that those risks are all wrong. The invasive-testing risks are currently a lot less than 1 in 200. With the noninvasive-screening option people can learn a lot more about their risk than is possible just based on age. So neither side of this "equation" is correct.

But, stepping back, there is a deeper problem. This recommendation assumes that everyone thinks that having a child with a chromosomal problem is exactly as bad as having a miscarriage. That's the logic under which comparing the probabilities is enough. This cannot be correct; it might not even be correct for the average person, and it's certainly not correct for *every* person. It seems extremely likely that for some women and families, they would much prefer to have a child with Down syndrome than to lose a healthy baby. Other women may feel that they are ill-equipped to deal with a special-needs child and, for them, that would be worse than a miscarriage. To just assume that these things are exactly equal for everyone seems very unrealistic.

If we go back to our decision-making framework from economics, this is like ignoring the personalized pluses-and-minuses part of the decision completely. It just makes no sense.

Increasingly, professional organizations and textbooks are moving away from the recommendation for 35-year-olds. They are now suggesting that all women be given the choice. But this doesn't necessarily translate into practice—in at least one recent survey, 92 percent of doctors routinely offered invasive testing to women over 35, and only 15 percent to women under 35.[18] If you *are* given the choice, the right decision depends on you.

Let's say you are 31 and you undergo the cell-free fetal DNA screening. With a good result on this, the baby's risk of having Down syndrome is around 1 in 100,000. The risk of miscarriage from the amniocentesis or CVS test is around 1 in 800. What you need to decide for yourself is whether having a baby with Down syndrome unexpectedly would be more than 125 times worse than having a miscarriage (that is, 100,000 divided by 800). If yes, then skip right to the invasive test—probably CVS given the timing. If no, then stick with the noninvasive screen. Of course, it's not easy to answer this question, but it *is* the question you need to answer.

Jesse and I spent a lot of time on this question (some of it even in person, not over e-mail). With Penelope, I ultimately decided to undergo the ultrasound screening and skip the invasive testing. The test went well, we stopped there, and Penelope was born healthy. In the end, I am not sure this was the right choice from a decision standpoint, and at some point later in the pregnancy I panicked that we should have done more accurate testing.

When I got pregnant with Finn I was sure the CVS testing was the right thing to do—I knew I had to know for sure with this pregnancy. In the language of the decision-theory above, relative to when I was expecting Penelope, our preferences had changed. The risk of a miscarriage seemed less important now that we already had one child. And the costs associated with a special-needs child seemed much higher.

But, in the end, the genetic counselor convinced me that the risks of CVS might have increased a lot given that they were so rarely performed. She pointed out that the cell-free fetal DNA testing was excellent—with a good test result, my risk was more like 1 in 35,000—and suggested this should be enough. We thought long and hard about it but decided—and I emphasize that this is a pretty unusual decision—that it still wasn't enough for us given our preferences.

In the end, I followed up the cell-free testing with an amniocentesis in the second trimester. We reasoned this was very low risk, and if we did it early there was still time to consider our options in the very unlikely event that the results showed something different from the cell-free testing. This worked well for us, although the genetic counselor (and my mother) thought it was very unusual. That's the thing about preferences, though: not everyone has the same ones.

The Surprising Perils of Gardening

have something to tell you. I noticed something about you today. I don't want you to get mad."

Jesse and I were getting ready for bed. I was just about four months pregnant. Jesse looked uncomfortable. I figured it must have been about how I looked. Was it finally time to move to maternity pants rather than just leaving my regular pants unbuttoned? Was my face getting puffy already? It turned out to be worse.

"You have a gray hair."

My first instinct was to pull it out, which I did. Then I panicked. What if it had friends? I immediately picked up the phone to call the hair salon. Jesse gently reminded me that (a) it was ten o'clock at night, and (b) you are not supposed to use hair dye during pregnancy. But, I argued, surely that restriction doesn't apply in such dire circumstances.

In the end, I was too lazy to schedule an appointment (although I did monitor carefully for any future appearances). But I knew there was likely to be a next time, and I'd probably have more gray hairs then.

The ban on hair dye is one of a number of restrictions that

aren't obvious from common sense. No hair dye, no hot tubs, no gardening? These can be hard to remember—in a few cases, I didn't even know that I should *think* to be concerned until after I did the activity. When Penelope was about seven months old, one of my Chinese colleagues expressed his surprise (and horror) that I hadn't worn a special vest during pregnancy to protect the baby from computer radiation. This is apparently all the rage in China; I had never even heard of it.

I scoffed at the antiradiation vest—there was obviously no evidence for it, and anyway, it was just a canvas vest. But, I wondered, what about the restrictions my doctors actually suggested? Were these just the American versions of the radiation vest?

Cat Litter and Gardening

I have a somewhat unpleasant cat named Captain Mittens. She terrorizes our cleaning lady and hisses at the nanny. Naturally, she is Penelope's favorite member of the household, so now we are stuck with her forever, if we weren't before. The Captain, as we call her, is all my fault. I brought her into the marriage, and I take care of her. Which includes cleaning the litter box. When I got pregnant I received a large number of e-mails (from my mother, my friend Nancy, etc.) with dire warnings about the cat: "Do not clean the litter box!" Sometimes with multiple exclamation points.

My doctor was kind of dismissive about this concern. She told me that if I didn't want the chore anymore, I could tell Jesse that it was dangerous, but in her view it was fine. I did briefly try to foist it on Jesse, but he wasn't buying. He'd do anything to protect the baby, but, as he constantly reminds me, the Captain isn't *his* cat. He wanted to know why, exactly, it was a problem for me to do this.

The worry about cat litter is toxoplasmosis. If that sounds familiar, it should: it comes up in the context of food restrictions, as the most common source of toxoplasmosis is uncooked meat. Recalling the discussion there: if you have been exposed to toxoplasmosis before pregnancy, there is no cause for concern, but if you are exposed for the first time during pregnancy, it can be dangerous for the baby, causing low IQ, vision problems, or death.

Although uncooked meat is the primary source of toxoplasmosis, it is also possible to get it from cat feces. If your cat has been eating uncooked meat, that is.

Despite the cat litter emphasis, the circumstances under which you can get this from a cat are fairly specific. Cats are infected by eating something (like raw meat) that gives them the parasite. The first time they are exposed they excrete the parasite eggs in their feces for several weeks; you can be infected through exposure to these. Once they are exposed once, they typically acquire immunity and are not exposed again. This means you're at risk if you're exposed to a cat during their *first* exposure. If your cat is old, regardless of whether it lives outside, it probably has already had this.

Perhaps for this reason, cat litter is not the main source of toxoplasmosis infection. In fact, in many studies it's not even a significant source of infection. For example, one study of pregnant women in Europe compared those with and without toxoplasmosis infection and looked to see what behaviors were more common among women who were infected.[1] They found no evidence that cats matter: women with this infection were no more likely to have a cat at all, clean a litter box, or have a cat who hunts outside. This might be puzzling given that we know it is *possible* to get this disease from cat feces. However, it seems likely that most people with cats do not let them hunt outside, or, if they do, their cats have already been exposed and have immunity.

The one caveat to this is that you may want to be a little careful if you get a kitten for the first time while pregnant, especially if you feed it a lot of raw meat. In fact, one study in the United States did find that owning three or more kittens (although not owning one or two) was associated with higher toxoplasmosis rates.[2] I can only imagine Jesse's face if I had suggested we get three (or more!) kittens while I was pregnant.

Somewhat surprisingly: although cat litter seems to have little risk, there is significant toxoplasmosis risk from *gardening*. That study in Europe that was reassuring on cats did find a strong association between toxoplasmosis and working with soil. This suggests that if you are planning to garden while pregnant you should use gloves, and possibly consider a mask to avoid inhaling any particles.

Forget about asking Jesse to clean the litter box; I should have been pushing him to plant the flowers.

Hair Dye

The primary concern with hair dye is that toxic chemicals in the dye will affect the baby. In very high doses, some of the chemical components of hair dye can increase birth defects in rodents. They can also cause cancer (again, in rats). This is a concern in principle, of course, but it is something of a stretch to compare the impact of directly injecting the pregnant rat with high doses of chemicals every day during pregnancy to three or four incidents of topical exposure (which is what you get from actually dyeing your hair).[3]

Human studies have generally not shown any association with an increased risk of birth defects. A couple of small studies have suggested a link with childhood cancer later, although larger studies have not confirmed this. Overall, the rat evidence doesn't seem to translate into a human link.[4]

In addition to birth defects and cancer, one study comparing Swedish hairdressers to the rest of the Swedish population showed a small but statistically significant increase in low-birth-weight babies among the hairdressers.[5] Because hairdressers work with hair dye more than the average person, this finding led to the concern that perhaps at high doses hair dye affects birth weight. In the end, this finding wasn't supported by other studies, and it seems likely that the result was driven by other aspects of the job (for example, the fact that hairdressers spend all of their time standing up).

There are a number of detailed reviews of this issue, and they all argue pretty compellingly that there is no reason to worry about hair dye use anytime in pregnancy.[6] In fact, even the American Congress of Obstetricians and Gynecologists suggests it's fine after the first trimester. To be fair, I think you probably should avoid injecting yourself with hair dye during the first trimester (or, really, at any time). Getting rid of a few gray hairs or touching up your roots is a different story.

Hot Tubs, Baths, Hot Yoga

As I was finishing this book I solicited comments from close friends: what did they really want to know about pregnancy? My friend Katie, who wasn't yet pregnant, was definitive: hot yoga. I told her that the book already covered regular yoga, but she was insistent: what about *hot* yoga. Was that a mistake?

It turns out that at least some hot yoga is frowned upon during pregnancy. This is for the same reason that very hot baths or extended periods in hot tubs are verboten: it has been suggested that raising your body temperature during the first months of pregnancy can lead to birth defects. Some evidence for this comes from a 2011 study.[7] The authors identified about 11,000 babies with birth defects and 7,000 without. They compared their mothers' behavior during pregnancy and looked at whether the mothers of the babies with birth defects were more likely to have used hot tubs during early pregnancy.

The authors considered seventeen birth defects. For two of them (an intestinal problem called gastroschisis and a neural tube defect called anencephaly) they found an association with hot tub use. On its own, it is a little hard to draw confident conclusions from this. Maybe these findings just showed up by chance because the authors were testing so many outcomes. However, other studies found the same effects on neural tube defects.[8] This connection is supported by animal studies, which can be done in a more controlled environment (researchers randomly heat up some pregnant animals and not others).

Altogether, this makes it seem quite likely that elevated temperature in the first trimester increases the risk of birth defects like spine bifida and anencephaly. This means that anything that elevates your temperature increases that risk: fever, hot tub use, very hot baths, and, yes, hot yoga.

It's probably important to note that the real concern is about an increase in body temperature to above 101 degrees or so. Hot tubs are typically about 105 degrees, as is Bikram Yoga. Spending time working out in a 105-degree environment can increase your body temperature. But a cooler hot tub or a cooler version of hot yoga (some are only 85 or 90 degrees) would be fine. In addition, the neural tube defect concern is limited to the first trimester; by the end of that period, neural tube formation is complete.

One question you might be asking yourself: What about really hot days? Is that the same thing? I wasn't able to unearth any studies about hot days and birth defects, but there is some evidence from Spain on the effect of heat on birth. The authors found that very hot days seemed to prompt women to go into labor earlier (by about 5 days).[9] It's possible that hot tubs or hot yoga later in pregnancy could have this effect also, although that's not something they cover in this study. The conclusion, perhaps, is that if it is 105 degrees out and you are 36 weeks pregnant, you should stay inside!

Safe Sex?

Many women wonder if it is safe to have sex during pregnancy. Is he hitting the baby? It turns out we don't really need research here; understanding the mechanics is enough. While you're pregnant the baby is inside a sac of fluid in the uterus, protected by the closed cervix. Having sex won't affect it at all; if you feel in the mood, go right ahead.

Two warnings, though. The cervix is a bit more sensitive during pregnancy, and if your partner hits it during intercourse you might bleed a bit; this is normal and not something to worry about at all. Second, as you get into later pregnancy, the good old missionary position isn't going to work as well. Creativity will be necessary!

Travel by Airplane

Prior to Penelope's arrival I traveled a fair amount, mostly for work. My first flight while pregnant was about 3 days after conception. My last was at 34 weeks, for a friend's birthday. Before the last trip I had to get a note from my doctor for fear they would turn me away at the gate: many airlines won't let you fly after 36 weeks. I think this is mostly because they are worried you might have the baby in the air.

But before 36 weeks there are typically no restrictions put on air travel by your doctor or by the airlines. The American Congress of Obstetricians and Gynecologists takes the view that air travel is fine. They suggest you wear your seat belt and, if necessary, get a seat belt extender (I narrowly avoided this on that last flight).

And despite this, people worry about radiation (maybe I should have been flying in a vest!).

You are exposed to cosmic radiation all the time, but when you fly the levels of radiation are higher than they are on the ground because there is less atmosphere to protect you. In general, there is a recommended limit on radiation exposure over the course of your pregnancy (technically, it's 1 mSv, but that probably has no more meaning for you than it does for me).

This is probably very conservative. Based on nonairline sources of radiation exposure (X-rays, for example), we do know that it can increase the risk of both miscarriage and birth defects, but only at exposure levels about 20 times higher than the recommended limit. There is some evidence, however, of an increased risk of childhood cancers at lower levels than this. One set of studies suggested that exposure to twice the recommended limit would increase the risk of offspring ever having a fatal cancer by 1 in 5,000.[10]

Unless you travel very frequently you are unlikely to reach even the most conservative limit for radiation exposure. One flight from Chicago to Boston would deliver about 1 percent of the limit. Long-haul international flights are worse: the longest available flight delivers about 15 percent of the limit. This might seem like a lot (if you take more than three round trips from New York to Tokyo you're over the limit), but it is worth noting that this is less than 1 percent of the level at which there is any actual demonstrated risk of birth defects or miscarriage. [11]

Consistent with this, at least one study that compared infant outcomes for women who did and did not fly during their pregnancies found no difference in preterm birth, fetal loss, or neonatal intensive care unit (NICU) admission.[12]

If you fly a lot for work—say, a couple of flights a week—or you are a flight attendant, it is possible that you would reach the 1 mSv radiation limit. In Europe, flight attendants are restricted to more limited routes during pregnancy to avoid this; in the United States there are no legal restrictions, but it may be prudent to limit exposure to some extent. If you are worried about your particular flights, the FAA Web site offers a way to calculate the radiation exposure from every flight, which you can use to calculate your total exposure.

What about the full body scanners at the airport? Again, these work with X-rays, and therefore entail some radiation exposure. These levels of exposure are quite small—maybe on the order of 0.01 percent of the 1 mSv limit—so they are probably not something to worry about. In practice, at least for the moment, most airports have normal metal detectors as well as the full body scan, and pregnant women are generally pointed toward the non-X-ray option. If you are worried, you can always opt for the pat down. It's not enjoyable, but it is radiation-free.

The Bottom Line

- Changing the cat litter is fine (make sure you wash your hands after) . . .

- . . . but gardening is associated with an increased risk of toxoplasmosis. It should be avoided.

- Dye away! Concerns about hair dye are overblown.

- Getting too hot during your first trimester—be it from a fever, a hot tub, or some type of superhot yoga—can lead to an increased risk of neural tube defects like spina bifida.

- Some airplane travel is completely fine. If you work on an airplane you might consider a modified schedule.

PART 3

The Second Trimester

. . .

. . .

Eating for Two? You Wish

As I was writing this book I talked to a lot of women who were pregnant, or had been pregnant—friends, family, my agent, colleagues. Almost without fail, the first thing they wanted to know was whether the book would cover weight gain during pregnancy. Everyone had a story about their doctor giving them a hard time about their weight, mostly about gaining too much. One woman actually told me she switched to a midwife after her doctor commented too frequently on her weight gain.

There is an enduring popular myth (held by almost every man I know, and many women who are not yet pregnant) of the pregnant woman who is eating for two. Women who spend their whole lives dieting, watching every calorie, arrive at pregnancy thinking it's the one time when they can just eat with abandon. And then reality sets in: not only is the amount you are supposed to gain restricted, but someone is literally monitoring and commenting on your weight every couple of weeks.

I didn't find weight to be such a big deal in the first trimester— like everyone else, I was too sick to eat much of anything—but around 12 or 14 weeks I started noticing I was getting a bit bigger.

Institute of Medicine Weight Gain Guidelines

Your suggested weight gain in pregnancy—at least by the standards of your doctor and the Institute of Medicine—varies with where you start. Here's a quick reference.

	Suggested Weight Gain (Pounds)
Underweight (BMI < 18.5)	28-40
Normal Weight (BMI 18.5-25)	25-35
Overweight (BMI 25-30)	15-25
Obese (BMI>30)	11-20

Why does it matter where you start? Think about it this way: if you are currently normal weight and not pregnant, doctors generally would suggest you keep your food intake the same. Add a pregnancy to the mix, and you need to eat a bit more (*not* twice as much, but about 300 or so more calories per day), which amounts to 25 to 35 pounds over the course of the pregnancy.

If you are overweight or obese and not pregnant, doctors would recommend you reduce your number of calories to lose weight. Add the same 300 pregnancy calories on top of that, and the total increase in calories is smaller. This amounts to gaining less than 25 to 35 pounds.

At some point I had to switch to my fat pants, and pretty soon those didn't fit either. I started to dread going to the doctor, as I knew there was a risk of a long lecture about my weight. Maybe it just felt this way, but it seemed like the standard second-trimester appointment entailed three minutes of actual baby monitoring and at least ten on weight-related issues: how much I had gained total, the rate of gain, was I really exercising, and so on.

The thing I found most frustrating about this was that I was really trying to do the right thing. I weighed myself carefully every Thursday morning, before eating anything, on a correctly calibrated digital scale. I watched what I was eating. After yet another lecture, I cut out sweets. I even made Jesse monitor me and keep me from eating dessert. This is definitely not something you want to make your husband do when you are pregnant.

I felt like I was actually doing pretty well. But the measurements from the doctor seemed random—sometimes agreeing with me and sometimes not. Between 17 and 20 weeks I gained 4 pounds according to my measurement, and nothing according to the doctor's. Then, between 20 and 24 weeks I gained 5 pounds by my measurement and 10 pounds by hers. This led to a long lecture—10 pounds in 4 weeks! Why was I sitting in front of the television eating chocolates all day?

I tried to explain that the 20-week measure must have been off, and even by her data, if you looked at the whole 17-to-24-week period I was actually doing fine. My OB listened and then put a little note in my file. I like to think that it said "Previous measurement in error," but it was probably more like "Belligerent and refuses to admit cookie abuse."

After that I started trying to game the system with my shoes. If I was feeling especially thin, I'd keep my shoes on during the weigh-in; if I was not, I'd take them off. If I weighed in at a high weight, I'd just say, "Oh, I guess I'm wearing my heavy shoes today!" This was surprisingly effective, although it seems like it probably shouldn't have been necessary.

But there is a deeper issue than the random measurement. I was never given a clear reason why I should worry. After all, I started out in a good place, in the normal BMI range. I later learned that despite all the monitoring and concern, more than half of women gain more weight than the recommended amount. Most of these women seem to look fine later, and have perfectly normal babies. So why was I avoiding those cookies?

Weight Gain and Later Weight: Yours, and Your Child's

Mom's Weight After Pregnancy

The first concern about weight gain is that if you put it on you have to take it off and, in the long run, being overweight is bad for your health. It is true that many women do have trouble losing weight after pregnancy and wind up retaining at least a few of those pregnancy pounds.

One study in the United Kingdom found that women who gained the recommended amount of weight during pregnancy ended up about 5 pounds heavier 6 months postpartum, and that those who gained more than the recommended amount ended up about 17 pounds heavier.[1] The good news is that this might be short-lived, at least for most women: a more recent study found that 90 percent of women who started out at normal weight had returned to a normal weight range by 24 months postpartum regardless of how much they gained during pregnancy.[2]

I don't think this bears much discussion. Why not? Well, for one thing, most of the research is not very informative. Retaining weight after pregnancy is closely related to being overweight or obese before pregnancy. But this means it is very hard for studies to separate out the impact of prepregnancy weight on later weight loss from the impact of pregnancy weight gain on later weight loss.

More important, we all try to lose weight now and then. You probably know how hard it is for you to do that. If you typically have an easy time losing weight, it'll probably be the same after the baby. If not, you may have a harder time. This is a book about having a healthy pregnancy and a healthy baby, not about weight loss. We'll leave that to another author, or at least another book.

Your Kid's Weight Later in Life

As the obesity "epidemic" has spread in the United States, some researchers have started to focus on the possibility that conditions in the womb contribute to childhood obesity. There is no question that obesity among young people has increased: around 20 percent of children and adolescents are currently obese, versus less than 5 percent in the 1960s.[3] Is it possible that higher rates of maternal weight gain during pregnancy have contributed to this increase? By eating those extra pancakes, are you dooming your child to a lifetime of dieting?

Maybe.

The main biological mechanism through which this might occur is insulin resistance. It's possible that excess weight gain during pregnancy could stimulate the fetus to produce more insulin, resulting in higher birth weight, limited sugar tolerance, and later weight gain. Researchers have shown that this actually does happen in mice, and they theorize that it might also happen in humans. However, it turns out to be difficult to show conclusively whether this is true for people. The correlation between childhood obesity and maternal weight gain is seen in a lot of studies. However, it's extremely difficult to show that they are *causally related*.

Let's be clear about what we are trying to figure out here. The decision I was making while pregnant was about how much weight to gain during pregnancy. This decision is unlikely to impact any other part of my daughter's life. It certainly won't change her genes, but it also is unlikely to change anything about how our family eats afterward, or how much money we spend on food, or how much exercise she gets. But all of these other things have huge impacts on childhood (and adult) obesity. Moreover, many of them are very closely related to weight gain in pregnancy.

Think about it this way: overweight women are more likely to gain in excess of the recommended amount of weight during pregnancy. And they are more likely to have overweight children. But is this because of the weight gain? Or is it because the eating habits that lead women to be overweight are the same that lead their children to be overweight? Or because Mom passes her metabolism on to her daughter? All plausible explanations, but only the first one is something you can change during pregnancy.

This basic problem makes it almost impossible to imagine how we might actually answer this question about weight gain and later-life obesity. Sure, a randomized trial would work great—let's recommend that some women gain a lot of weight and some gain almost none—but we are going to again run into problems on our ethics review. Without this, our best bet is to sort among studies to try to find the best ones, with the caveat that nothing is going to be *really* convincing.

One of the best papers on this comes from an extremely long-term study of 2,500 Danish children born between 1959 and 1961.[4] This study started with 4,200 mothers, and around the time of their children's births collected information on prepregnancy weight and weight gain during pregnancy, along with a few other variables. The researchers followed at least some of the children until the present: the paper was published in 2010 and included data on offspring BMI all the way up to age 42! (A reminder: BMI is weight in kilograms divided by height in meters squared; 18 to 25 is "normal").

At every age the authors looked at, BMI was higher for people whose mothers gained more weight in pregnancy. On average, for every kilogram Mom gained, BMI increased by about 0.03, and this continued through adulthood. This study is pretty good, and the ability to follow people through adulthood is neat. Of course, it is not without its problems. For one thing, the ranges of weight gain are very small: the upper end of the range in this study is more than 35 pounds, and a relatively small percentage of people gain in that range. What happens if you gain 80 pounds during pregnancy? You're not going to learn the answer to that here. There is also the obvious issue: there are some differences across women to begin with, which could be what produced these results.

But let's say we take these conclusions at face value: it seems that gaining more weight increases your child's weight later. However, this effect is tiny. If you gain 10 pounds over the recommendation during pregnancy, you would increase your child's expected BMI by about 0.13. If your child is 5 feet 6 inches, this is an increase in weight from 149 to 150 pounds. That's before versus after breakfast, at least for me.

There are other studies that show similar results. Weight gain matters, yes, but the changes are small. A pound or two here or there. [5, 6, 7]

In the end, I wasn't especially convinced that any of the studies of this showed causal evidence. But even if these effects *were* causal, it didn't seem to matter. The effects were tiny. On the

The Bottom Line

- What you put on you have to take off (at least if you want to get back to pre-pregnancy condition). Most women are able to do this, although it takes a few months (don't pressure yourself).

- Impacts of weight gain on child weight later are extremely small if they are there at all.

scale of everything else I am likely to do to impact my child's weight, this just wasn't very important.

Where It Really Makes a Difference: Weight Gain and Birth Weight

Worrying about the long-term effect of pregnancy weight gain probably isn't worth it. But weight could still matter for the short term. In fact, it does matter in one significant way: weight gain during pregnancy relates very closely to your baby's birth weight. The more weight you gain, the larger your baby is likely to be *relative to the timing of his birth*.

All else being equal, the longer the baby sticks around in your womb, the larger he will be. A baby born at 42 weeks will be larger than he would have been if he were born at 37 weeks. This is normal, and typically fine: there are a wide range of healthy weights for babies, from less than 6 pounds to well over 10 pounds.

More concerning to doctors is when a baby is very small or very large relative to its time spent in the womb; babies in either of these categories are at higher risk for various complications: breathing problems, insulin resistance, and heart problems, among others. Babies who are very large relative to the amount of time in the womb are termed *large for gestational age* (LGA); babies who are very small are termed *small for gestational age* (SGA).

Baby birth weight is related to pregnancy weight gain. If you go too far outside the weight gain guidelines, you are increasingly likely to have a baby who is either LGA or SGA.

This is well known, and has been for a long time. When my *mormor* (Swedish for grandmother) was pregnant with my mom, she was told to keep her weight gain to a minimum. This would keep the baby small and make delivery easier. She followed this advice, and my mom was only about 6 pounds at birth. It's not clear whether this advice is so great; she also received the advice that breast-feeding was only for poor immigrants, which (fortunately for my mother!) she actually was.

It's also easy to see the weight-gain–baby-weight connection in data. In the United States, weight gain during pregnancy is often recorded on infant birth certificates, and studies of this show a strong association with birth weight. Consider a recent study of about 500,000 births in Florida.[8] The study divided women by weight gain, and the graph below shows the chance of an abnormally large or small baby for women who gained the recommended amount of weight, 10 pounds too little and 10 pounds too much.

Weight Gain, Large Babies, and Small Babies

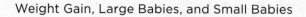
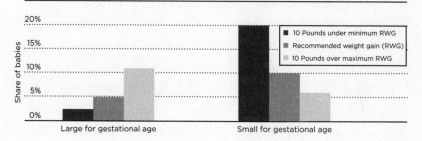

This graph uses data from the normal-weight women in the study, but the pattern was exactly the same for women who started overweight or underweight.

Relative to those who gain the recommended amount, women who gain less than what's recommended are less likely to have babies who are large for gestational age, but more likely to have babies who are small. On the other hand, those who gain more than recommended are more likely to have abnormally large babies and less likely to have small ones.

These effects are big. I started my pregnancy at around 150 pounds. If I gained in the recommended range (25 to 35 pounds), my chance of having an abnormally large baby was about 5 percent, and my chance of having an abnormally small baby was around 10 percent. If I gained 10 pounds *less* than was recommended (ha! not likely), my chance of having a really large baby would have been cut in half, but my chance of having a very small baby would have doubled. On the other hand, if I gained 10 pounds more, I would have been only about half as likely to have a very small baby but twice as likely to have a very large one.

This study, like most studies of this issue, focused on broad categories: gain less than recommended, gain the recommended amount, or gain more than recommended. This might make you think that there is something magical about going over or under the guidelines, even by just a pound (in fact, some doctors and nurses treat these guidelines like this). Most things in biology don't work this way, and pregnancy weight is no exception. A weight gain of 36 pounds and 35 pounds are really, really similar. It is *not* the case that the moment you gain 36 pounds the risks instantly change.

Although 36 (or 24) pounds is not a magic number, it is hard to avoid the conclusion that, in general, weight gain is related to baby size, and that going far outside the recommendations does change the baby's size. But so what? What are the risks to very small or large babies?

Small for Gestational Age (SGA): SGA babies are usually defined as those in the bottom 10 percent in terms of birth weight relative to their time in the womb; some studies take a more extreme definition and use only babies in the bottom 2.5 percent in terms of birth weight. Although babies in this group are often fine, especially if they are born at full term, they are much more likely to have complications. A study in Finland[9] found that 42 percent of SGA babies had some complications. These included difficulty breathing, difficulty regulating blood sugar, and abnormal neurological signs. For babies who are born prematurely, being small for gestational age is more serious. A recent study from Greece showed that mortality rates are much higher for SGA babies than for those who are appropriate for gestational age, and they are at risk for serious lung complications.[10] Some studies suggest that babies who are born SGA have more long-term issues, including a higher risk for diabetes and lower cognitive skills.[11]

Large for Gestational Age (LGA): Babies in the top 10 percent in terms of birth weight are classified as large for gestational age. Women with gestational diabetes often have LGA babies; gestational diabetes causes its own set of complications. For women who are not diabetic, the most significant complication associated with LGA babies is difficulty in delivery, including an increased chance of requiring a C-section and an increased risk of instrument-assisted delivery.[12, 13]

On average, the complications associated with a very small baby are much more serious than those associated with a very large baby. If you had to choose, most women would prefer to face the increased risk of a C-section rather than an increased risk of breathing problems or neurological complications for their baby. **On its own, this probably means that you should be more concerned about gaining too little weight than too much weight.**

That statement is based only on the baby-size evidence. What about other outcomes? One particular concern is prematurity— the risk that over or under gaining might increase the chance of having a premature baby.

The evidence on this is mixed. It is actually somewhat difficult to evaluate, for a simple reason: the longer you are pregnant, the more weight you gain. If you gave birth at 32 weeks, you naturally gained less than someone who gave birth at 40 weeks. But this isn't because too little weight gain is associated with preterm birth! In addition, there are medical conditions that cause you to gain more or less weight, and which themselves are associated with preterm birth (for example, gestational diabetes).

Given both of these problems, it's not surprising that it's hard to be conclusive. In a large study of about 33,000 births in New York,[14] authors were able to relate the risk of having a birth before 37 weeks to the amount of weight gained. For women who started out normal weight, the risk of prematurity was similar for any weight gain between 22 and 45 pounds. However, those who gained less than 22 pounds or more than 45 pounds had a higher rate of preterm birth (about 1.3 to 1.5 times as high). Overweight or obese women who gained more than 45 pounds had a much higher rate of preterm birth (as much as 70 percent higher).

This study points to risks from *either* too much or too little weight gain; other studies have tended to find this relationship only for too little weight gain.[15, 16] In either case, the impact seems to be small; it isn't clear whether this adds much to our concerns.

So, Are the Recommendations Right?

This evidence was strong enough to convince me that weight gain *does matter* in the sense that it impacts the baby's size in particular. But that wasn't quite the same as convincing me that the weekly haranguing was appropriate. How should I think about the downside to gaining too much weight? How should I trade that off against the fact that, let's face it, I was hungry and I like cookies.

The one overwhelming thing I took away from this was that it doesn't matter very much. Gaining a few pounds, even 10 or 15, over the weight limit is not very important. Even in studies that do find some risks to too much weight gain, these effects are small and don't kick in for women who gain, say, 37 pounds. At one visit I was informed that if I continued my current rate of gaining, I would be at 36 pounds, and the limit was 35, so I should try to cut down. Nothing—not evidence and not basic logic—supports this.

So, basically, relax.

When we start talking about *a lot* more or less than the recommendation, it seems clear that the downsides to a very small baby are worse than those to a very large baby. I was, in the end, kind of surprised that the doctor made such a big deal about the weeks when I gained too much weight, and never said anything during the weeks when I gained nothing.

As I thought more about this, I wondered whether these recommendations that everyone is so obsessed with are even *right*. I thought about how the recommendations were made. Looking at the numbers carefully, it became clear that they were made with the goal being to maximize the chance of having a "normal for gestational age" baby (i.e., not too large or too small).

If I gained 30 pounds, right in the middle of the recommended amount, the chance of *either* a too-small or too-big baby was 15 percent. If I gained 40 pounds, it was 18 percent. If I gained only 20 pounds, it was 23 percent. So my best bet for a normal-size baby was 30 pounds of weight gain.

But thinking about it just half a second more, this logic seemed flawed. The complications associated with a very small baby are, on average, more severe than those associated with a very large baby. But the guidelines seemed to be focused on minimizing the total number of too-large or too-small babies.

At a weight gain of 30 pounds we'd expect 10 percent of women to have very small babies and 5 percent to have very large babies. At a weight gain of 40 pounds, these figures are 7 percent and 11 percent. Yes, there is an increase in very large babies, but there is a decrease in very small ones. But because a very small baby is worse in terms of complications, is this maybe actually better?* In order to really make the right recommendation, we

---

* One reason it might not be is if normal-size babies are far, far better than either extreme. In this case we could argue for focusing only on getting as many of those as possible. In practice, this is probably not accurate.

need to think about what recommendation does the best job limiting the actual *complications*. And in this particular case, that might well be an argument for increasing the recommended weight gain, at least by a few pounds.

So what happened to me? In the end, I gained 30.3 pounds— from 149.0 to 179.3 (after all the lecturing, I had gotten very, very precise about measurement). They actually weighed me for a final time when we arrived at the hospital, I suppose just to see whether I'd binged on ice cream after the weigh-in at the doctor's office that morning. All I can say is it is a good thing they didn't try to give me a hard time about it in the middle of a contraction—after all, they hadn't given me time to remove my shoes!

The Bottom Line on Weight

- On average, if you gain more weight, your baby will be larger. If you gain less weight, your baby will be smaller.

- Both very large and very small babies face additional risks, although too-small babies face greater risks. If anything, you should probably be more concerned about gaining too little weight than too much.

- But, mostly, chill out.

. . .

Pink and Blue

Very early on in pregnancy—maybe even at my seven-week ultrasound—I got a report on the speed of Penelope's pulse. On average, fetal heart rates are much faster than adults'. A typical number would be in the range of 120 to 160 or so. Penelope was around 150, which is on the faster end. My mother-in-law, Joyce, immediately stated that the baby was a girl. *For sure.*

Her story was that girls have a faster fetal heart rate. Her doctor used this system to figure out the gender of both of her kids. He got it right both times. Jesse was excited; he really wanted a girl.

It was many weeks between this first ultrasound and when we actually did learn that Penelope was a girl. In this time, Jesse dug up a paper on fetal heart rate and gender. The authors collected data from 500 women, about half of whom had a girl and half a boy. The average female heart rate was 151.7 and the average male heart rate was 154.9. These were not significantly different (if anything, the male heart rates were *higher*, contrary to Joyce's theory). The paper concluded, "Contrary to beliefs commonly held by many pregnant women and their families (*I'm looking at you, Joyce*), there are no significant differences between male and female fetal heart rate during the first trimester."[1]

Jesse sent along an e-mail about this. Joyce was skeptical. "All I'm saying is that my doctor was right both times. So there must be something to it."

No, we insisted, these guys used 500 people—500 data points versus her 2—and showed that there was no connection. We never really convinced her, and our case wasn't really helped when she turned out to be right.

In fact, fetal heart rate notwithstanding, there are a number of ways to learn the sex of your baby before birth.

If you do a CVS test in the first trimester (or an amniocentesis later), you can learn the baby's sex at that point. Because chromosomes differ for boys and girls (an XY for a boy versus two Xs for a girl), this is part of the genetic mapping.

If you forgo this test you can still learn your baby's sex on an ultrasound. For many people (us included) this happened around 20 weeks.

It's at this point that many doctors will do a "midtrimester" ultrasound. The baby is sufficiently developed at this point that you can look at all kinds of things—how well the blood is flowing through the heart, the number of fingers and toes, location of organs, and so on—and, of course, genitals.

Although the 20-week ultrasound is common, it's actually possible to see fetal sex on an ultrasound as early as 12 weeks, especially if it is a boy. By 15 or 16 weeks you can typically tell either way. Of course, because learning your baby's sex is not actually a medical necessity, most doctors will not do an additional ultrasound to figure it out. You'll just have to wait or, if you are really going crazy wondering, you can go to a private ultrasound clinic. I did briefly consider this when my curiosity got overwhelming.

If you really, really can't wait, you're in luck. Within the last few years researchers have made a lot of progress on determining fetal sex from a maternal blood sample. In principle, this can be done pretty much as soon as you're pregnant. The testing relies on the fact that your blood mingles with your baby's (to a small extent) and, therefore, in every sample of Mom's blood there are some fetal cells.

If the fetus is a boy, these cells contain a Y chromosome. You, as the pregnant woman, definitely *do not* have any Y chromosomes. To greatly simplify, these tests rely on looking for a signal of a Y chromosome in Mom's blood. If evidence of one is found, it's a boy. If not, it's probably a girl. I say "probably" because the lack of a Y chromosome could also be explained by not having picked up any of the baby's cells.

This technology is relatively new, but it's pretty effective. In one study from 2010, researchers collected blood from 201 women. In 10 cases their results were inconclusive. In 77 the result was "girl," and in 71 of those cases the baby was a girl (of the other cases, 4 ended in miscarriage and 2 had unknown gender). In 112 cases the result was "boy," and in 105 of those cases the baby was a boy (of the others, there were 5 miscarriages and 2 babies with unknown gender).[2]

At the moment, this test isn't something you would ask for just because you want to know your baby's sex. It's more commonly used for clinical purposes. For example, families in which there is a genetic disease associated with the Y chromosome would want to know early on if their child is a boy, which would necessitate further testing. However, increasing moves toward commercializing this mean that within a few years it's likely to be accessible to those parents who just cannot wait to get the gender-specific shopping started.

Jesse and I were dying to find out the sex of the baby. We couldn't imagine waiting until she was born. When they finally did tell us, Jesse was so excited to tell everyone we knew that he abandoned me in the doctor's office to go outside and send a text (there was no phone service in the office with the ultrasound). Not everyone feels this way. Surveys find that around half, or slightly more, of couples choose to learn the sex of the baby.[3]

Even if you don't want to know, or don't plan to find out, it's hard not to guess. It's even harder to get people not to guess. Random people will stop you on the street to say things like, "Oh, I know you must be carrying a boy, your belly is so high/low/big/small." We already debunked the fetal heart rate. Is there any truth to any of these old wives' tales?

I looked hard in the medical literature, but apparently doctors have better things to do than research whether belly position predicts fetal sex. I couldn't find anything—nothing to confirm or deny. I took this to mean that none works especially well. Of course, they all work about 50 percent of the time; presumably this is how Joyce's doctor managed to get it right—with two pregnancies, he had a 25 percent chance of being correct both times, even with random guessing!

Once you're pregnant it's too late to impact the sex of the baby. You can find out early, or find out later, but you can't do anything to change it. But you might wonder—many people do—whether you can do anything about this before conception. I have one friend who really, really wanted her first child to be a girl. She asked me at some point—was there anything she could do to achieve that?

If you are really serious about it, the answer is yes. Various invasive technologies can increase your chances of having a girl or boy baby. There is something called *sperm sorting*, in which your partner's sperm are sorted, and only some of them—the ones with the right gender—are used in artificial insemination. This has a high, although definitely not perfect, success rate. If you're doing in vitro fertilization, it can in principle be combined with something called *preimplantation genetic diagnosis* to select only male or female embryos.

But let's assume that you're not committed enough to move to assisted reproductive technologies to get the gender you want. In lieu of this, there's a traditional method—the Shettles Method— that purports to use the timing of sex to get the gender you want. The theory is as follows: Y chromosome sperm (those that would produce a boy) are fast swimmers but they die off quickly; X chromosome sperm (those that would produce a girl) are slower swimmers but they last longer.

Therefore, if you want to have a girl, you should have sex several days before ovulation (but *not* right at ovulation). Then, when you do ovulate, the boy-producing sperm have died, and the girl-producing sperm are waiting. If you want to have a boy, you should have sex right at ovulation. Because the boy-producing sperm are faster, they'll rush up to the egg and win.

There is no evidence that this works. In a 1995 study in the *New England Journal of Medicine* researchers reported on a cohort of women followed for months as they tried to conceive (we also referred to this study in the discussion of conception). There was no relationship between the timing of sex in relation to ovulation and the gender of the offspring.[4] Sorry, you'll just have to take your chances.

The Bottom Line

- If you want to learn your baby's sex before birth, you can do so through CVS, amniocentesis, or ultrasound.

- There's no affirmative evidence that fetal heart rate or other old wives' tales do a good job of predicting gender.

- You cannot increase your chances of a particular gender by changing the timing of sex before conception.

Working Out and Resting Up

The women I know varied in how uncomfortable they found their pregnancies (although almost no one I know felt that the second trimester was "magical" or "glowing"). But without exception the two areas that everyone ultimately found problematic were exercise and sleep. As you get bigger and bigger, it's just hard to keep doing either of these normally. I actually do have one friend whom I saw jogging when she was 41 weeks pregnant. Hats off to you, lady. I had to quit running at 5 months, and by the end even walking on the treadmill was really uncomfortable. I admit to being repeatedly tempted to cut out the exercising. I also started to wonder, as I got bigger and bigger and bigger, whether it might actually be a problem. On the one hand, my doctor asked me every time I saw her whether I was still exercising and emphasized how important that was. On the other hand, I knew certain conditions could be exacerbated by exercise. I wondered if maybe I was overdoing it (Jesse assures me that, having seen how fast I was going on the treadmill, I could not possibly have been overdoing it). So what was it? Is exercise really important? Or dangerous? Or both?

Let's start with the most basic fact: for the most part, exercising more leads to slightly less weight gain during pregnancy. Hopefully this is not a surprise. One reason most of us work out when not pregnant is to stay in shape, or lose weight. If you burn 300 calories on the treadmill, that's 300 more calories you can eat. A lot of things change during pregnancy, but the basic calories-in-calories-out rule does not.

Logic dictates that this would be true, and we can see it in randomized trials. Because of concerns about excess weight gain during pregnancy, there are a number of studies that try to encourage women to exercise in the hope that they will stay comparatively svelte. On average, this seems to work. In a 2010 review paper, researchers identified 12 randomized trials of various types of exercise.[1] Most studies involved walking, water aerobics, or cycling, usually about three times a week.

On average, women who were encouraged to exercise gained about 1.3 fewer pounds during their pregnancies than women who were not. That figure is statistically significant, but it's small. This is probably not a big surprise to those of us who have tried to lose weight through exercise. You just don't burn that many calories when you work out, at least not relative to eating. This is true even when you are working out at normal, nonpregnancy levels, and it's only more true for the type and intensity of exercise most of us are able to do while pregnant. By the end of my pregnancy, I felt really great that I was still walking for about thirty minutes on the treadmill on most (okay, some) days. However, given the speed, this amounted to about 170 calories, the equivalent of the bowl of cereal I often ate at three A.M.

In principle, exercising while pregnant could have other benefits. A 2009 review article[2] summarized all of the existing randomized trials of exercise programs that reported effects on things *other than* weight gain, like baby size, preterm birth, etc. This article is comprehensive, but ultimately disappointing in its evidence. In fact, the authors say at the start: "Overall, the trials are quite small, and none are of high methodological quality." In other words, we don't know much.

What we do learn is that, at least in these small studies, exercise doesn't seem to have much of an impact on anything. No change in preterm birth, or gestational age, or rate of C-section, or fetal growth. There is no evidence of a difference in baby APGAR scores or in the length of labor.

So there is not a lot of reason to start exercising. There is also no reason to stop. The same randomized studies that show no clear benefits of exercise also show no downsides. In fact, on average, when you compare women who exercise to those who do not, the ones who exercise do seem to have lower-risk pregnancies. Of course, this is almost certainly because they are healthier to begin with, but it reinforces the view that there is no reason to stop exercising.

Exercising in general is fine; but are there any exercises you *shouldn't* do? There are definitely some pregnancy complications (placenta previa, for example) for which doctors encourage women to limit or eliminate exercise. But what about those of us lucky enough to have a healthy, uncomplicated pregnancy?

The biggest prohibition is on normal sit-ups or crunches, where you lie flat on your back. Usually these are prohibited after 20 weeks. Why? For the same reason you are not supposed to lie flat on your back when you sleep—the possibility of restricted blood flow. More on this below. But the bottom line is that for most women this is fine, and you'd know if it wasn't fine for you because it would be uncomfortable. If you can do a sit-up, even after 20 weeks, go right ahead.

One thing I will say: in the interest of science, at 34 weeks pregnant I tried a full sit-up with absolutely no luck. At some point, nature may force you into this restriction, whether you like it or not.

A second issue, also related to abdominal exercises, is something called *diastasis recti abdominis*: separation of the abdominal muscles. This happens to a very large percentage of pregnant women (you'll know if it happens to you). It usually goes back to normal after pregnancy. A number of Web sites will tell you that if this happens you should stop all abdominal exercises. In the literature, I can find no support for this claim. In fact, at least one randomized (but small) study suggests that continuing to work the abdominals actually makes this condition better, not worse.[3] Again, if you feel up to it, just keep going.

Really, are there *any* exercises you should avoid? The answer is, of course, yes. Exercise in which physical trauma is possible or likely (e.g., tackle football) should probably be avoided. Your baby is actually pretty well protected by the womb, but common sense suggests that there may be a limit. For some of the same reasons, doctors tend to recommend that you avoid activities like skiing or rock climbing, where falling is possible; most women have some trouble with balance during pregnancy, which makes falling more likely. A fall while skiing could possibly cause the placenta to detach, which is a very serious complication.

There is also some evidence that exercising really hard during pregnancy could (very temporarily, during the period of exercise) compromise blood flow to the baby. In one study of Olympic-level athletes, researchers found that when women exercised so hard that they pushed their heart rate to more than 90 percent of their maximum, there was some decreased blood flow to the baby.[4] If you are a serious athlete, pregnancy might not be the ideal time to try to achieve your personal best in a marathon. This is probably not applicable to the vast majority of us who struggle to get in those two- or three-mile runs a few times a week.

It's one thing to think about continuing your regular exercise during pregnancy. It's another to think about *adding* pregnancy-specific exercises to the routine. The very idea is exhausting.

Having said this, labor is basically a really long workout that you can't quit in the middle of. So maybe you should be preparing specifically for that. In fact, the uterus actually *is* preparing itself by flexing and unflexing—that's what Braxton Hicks contractions are. You aren't going to be able to do much to help it along, but there are two particular things you can do: Kegels and prenatal yoga.

Kegels

Kegels get a lot of play in the world of pregnancy. In medical terms, these are called pelvic floor exercises. Here's how to find your pelvic muscles if you haven't already. Go pee (shouldn't be too hard, given that you are pregnant). Squeeze your muscles to stop midstream. Feel that? Those are your pelvic floor muscles (men have these, too; same procedure to find them). Kegels are nothing more than exercises where you repeatedly squeeze those muscles to strengthen them.

Women's magazines sometimes recommend you work on these muscles even when not pregnant, so that you can use them during sex. Indeed, this is a common "treatment" for female sexual dysfunction (i.e., inability to orgasm), although hard empirical evidence on its effectiveness is lacking.[5] However, it does turn out that strengthening these muscles *during pregnancy* has several benefits.

Nearly all women experience some urinary incontinence during late pregnancy or after delivery—most commonly when sneezing or coughing. Some women experience more severe forms—they pee when laughing, during strenuous exercise, etc.—and this can continue for significant periods—years, even—postpartum. Kegels are extremely good for preventing this.

There are many studies of this, but let's take one typical one, which was run in Taiwan and published in 2011.[6] It was a randomized trial: 300 women were recruited; 150 were assigned to do Kegel exercises and the other 150 were left to their own devices. The particular exercise was fairly standard: twice a day, women did 3 sets of 8 Kegels, where they tightened and held for 6 seconds, with 2-minute breaks between each set. This is not that much; it amounts to maybe 15 or 20 minutes a day total.

Women in this study were asked to complete a 6-item questionnaire at several points during their pregnancy and right after. The questions focused on urinary control: e.g., how often do you pee, and do you experience urine leakage at various times. Each question was worth 1 point, with a maximum score of 6, which would indicate very bad urinary symptoms. Lower scores were better. The graph below shows scores on this questionnaire for women in the Kegels group and those in the control group at various points during their pregnancies.

Kegels and Urinary Incontinence

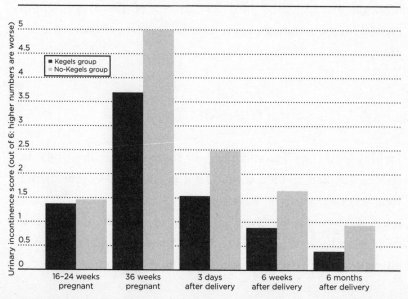

These women were very similar early in their pregnancies (before they started the exercises), but differences emerged at the end of their pregnancies and continued up to 6 months postdelivery. Women who do Kegels regularly are significantly less likely to have urinary leakage. Of course, this is just like any other exercise: it works by building up your muscles. So there is no reason not to start even before you are pregnant, although these studies show you can get the benefits of the exercise even if you start midway through the pregnancy.

This study shows results similar to a number of others. A review article from 2009 suggests that women who are encouraged to do these exercises are less than half as likely as control women to experience any urinary incontinence during late pregnancy or in the postpartum period.[7] This is especially true for women having their first baby.

And there might be more: at least one small randomized study[8] focused on the birth experience of women encouraged to do Kegels and those who were not. Women in the Kegels group spent a slightly shorter time pushing (40 minutes versus 45 minutes, on average), and only 22 percent of the Kegels group pushed for more than an hour, versus 37 percent of the no-Kegels group.

Prenatal Yoga

I wish I liked yoga. I would like to be someone who likes yoga. In college, I signed up for a semester's worth of classes at the gym. I went to one class. Jesse still asks when I'm going to go back for the rest. I went to hot yoga once, passed out during class, and never went back. When I first got my iPhone, I bought a yoga app. I used it—you guessed it—one time, when I was locked out of my house waiting for someone to come home and let me in. Basically, I like the idea of yoga, but hate actually doing it.

I was especially upset about my dislike of yoga during pregnancy, because there is actually some evidence that prenatal yoga is beneficial on a variety of dimensions. This is not a very well-researched area; the studies tend to be small, and a lot of the outcomes are things like "self-actualization," which is probably very important but is awfully difficult to quantify. In addition, the people running these studies often seem to really like yoga, so there is a feeling that maybe their biases are coloring their results. On the other hand, there are a few positive concrete outcomes, and the advantage of a randomized study is that it's relatively hard to manipulate.

One study of about 90 women in Taiwan showed that the women randomly assigned to a 12-week yoga program experienced a reduction (from 43 percent to 38 percent) in discomfort in the last couple of weeks of pregnancy.[9] A similar intervention in Thailand focused on 74 women, and measured labor pain and labor duration.[10] In this study, the women in the yoga group reported lower levels of pain at several different times during labor, and much shorter first-stage (i.e., before pushing) labor. The effects on labor length were actually huge in this study: labor was two and a half hours shorter for the yoga group.

Both of these studies were small, and there are not a lot of others to rely on, so it is hard to be enormously confident in the conclusions here. It is also not clear why this would work. More flexibility? Opening up the pelvis? Who knows. For whatever reason, the word on yoga is positive. So positive, in fact, that I even considered trying it. Once.

The Bottom Line

- General exercise during pregnancy is fine. Not exercising during pregnancy is also fine. By and large, you should feel comfortable continuing to do what you are already doing.

- Kegels prevent urinary incontinence and quite possibly improve your pushing ability in labor. Do them.

- Prenatal yoga is definitely worth trying. Although the studies are not large, they do show some large effects. If nothing else, perhaps you will improve your self-actualization.

Insomnia

As far as I can tell, sleeping normally during pregnancy is basically impossible. Despite the body pillows, extra blankets, and, in extreme cases, exiling one's husband to the guest room, by the end it's almost impossible to get through the night. I once got a text from my friend Heather when she was 29 weeks pregnant at 3:58 A.M.: "I've got several small stuffed sheep ready to go. To which god must I sacrifice these things to get a little sleep?"

Adding insult to injury, by the time you get to 20 weeks of pregnancy, your sleep position is significantly restricted. At my 20-week visit, my OB reminded me: no more sleeping on my back, and ideally I should stay on my left side. I tried to follow this rule, but it made things even more difficult. I awoke several times late in pregnancy to find my left leg completely asleep (at least *it* was getting some rest).

In my normal nonpregnant state I would treat insomnia with Unisom or Tylenol PM. And I'd never sleep on my side. Was I really helping my baby by lying uncomfortably and avoiding drugs?

Sleep Aids: The most commonly used over-the-counter medication for sleep is Unisom. If this works for you, go for it. It's a pregnancy Category B drug, meaning it's widely used and there is no evidence of risk to your baby (more on drug categories in the next chapter).

Unisom doesn't work for everyone. What about something stronger? Ambien is an obvious option. The evidence on Ambien safety is good, but not as unequivocal as it is for Unisom. A number of studies in humans have shown occasional Ambien use to be safe.[11] A caution is that there is at least one study, in Taiwan, that demonstrated that women who had long-term prescriptions for Ambien during pregnancy were more likely to have preterm and low-birth-weight babies.[12]

Sleep Position: You're not supposed to sleep on your back. The theory is that as the uterus gets larger (beyond 20 weeks or so), it can compress an important blood vessel. This decreases Mom's blood pressure, and can reduce blood flow to the placenta and the baby. That this occurs is something we know from physiology. What is the more relevant question for you is whether there is any evidence that this actually has risks for the baby. If you wake up on your back, should you worry?

As it turns out, very likely not.

There are various ways you can try to figure this out. Because there is a clear biological mechanism, the most obvious way is to try to see if that mechanism really works the way that is claimed. In one very nice study of this, researchers made women lie on their backs and measured the blood flow to the uterus. They found that lying down has no particularly bad impact on blood flow. A couple of women in that study became uncomfortable, but felt better when they changed positions. The authors concluded that some women might be uncomfortable sleeping on their backs, but if you are not one of them, you should feel fine about it. [13]

This paper was included as part of a review article about the topic. Their conclusion, which I think is clear and succinct, is as follows:

> Advising women to sleep or lie exclusively on the left side is not practical and is irrelevant to the vast majority of patients. Instead, women should be told that a small minority of pregnant women feel faint when lying flat. Women can easily determine whether lying flat has this effect on them, and most will adopt a comfortable position that is likely to be a left supine position or variant thereof . . . since finding a comfortable position in bed in late pregnancy is not easy, physicians should refrain from providing impractical advice.[14]

The above review concluded that the no-back-sleeping recommendation doesn't make sense. When I was making this decision with Penelope, that was where the bulk of the evidence lay. However, a recent study has questioned this, and deserves some discussion. It shows a scary link between maternal sleep position and stillbirth.[15]

The method in this study is straightforward. The researchers identified women who had a recent stillbirth, and interviewed them about their behaviors while pregnant. They also spoke to some women who had healthy babies. The idea was to look for what behaviors differed between the two groups, and then conclude that those behaviors might have contributed to the stillbirths.

It turns out that sleeping on the back or the right side was associated with a higher rate of stillbirth. The effect is large: the stillbirth rate was about twice as high for women sleeping on their backs. This study wasn't perfect. The sample size was small and the researchers were testing a lot of different theories, not just sleep position.

Having said this, there isn't anything obviously *wrong* with the paper that would lead one to fully discount the conclusions. We're left in a frustrating but common position when it comes to academic debates: more research is needed. In the interim, it's not clear what the right conclusion is. Sleeping on your left side is unlikely to be bad, so that's a good option if you can manage to get to sleep that way.

For me, one of the most infuriating things about the insomnia was when people would tell me things like, "You think you are tired now! Wait until the baby comes!" And it is unfortunately true: however little sleep you are getting at the end of pregnancy, you'll probably get less once the baby arrives. But there is a silver lining: when you do finally get a chance to sleep, there are none of those pregnancy aches and pains that kept you up. The quality of sleep goes up a lot, even if the quantity does not.

The Bottom Line

- Unisom is safe to take. Ambien is also probably safe, but the evidence is a bit more mixed.

- Most evidence suggests that restrictions on back sleeping are overblown, although one recent study disagrees. Concrete guidance is limited.

. . .

Drug Safety

am lucky to be generally healthy (my mother likes to take credit, saying it's due to her policy of exposing me to a lot of germs as a child). I don't get a lot of colds, and I never get the flu. A few years ago Jesse actually got pneumonia, and I never even had a cough. I do, however, have one weakness: urinary tract infections. If you've ever had one of these, you will know why this is a serious problem. It's like a combination of a stomach flu and someone kicking you in the crotch.

I had heard that these were more common during pregnancy, which terrified me, but in the end I managed to avoid getting one until I was almost six months along. And then, while visiting my family for Christmas, I woke up at three A.M. to the familiar feeling of discomfort, knowing it would get worse if I didn't treat it soon.

As it happens, I carry around two drugs to treat this: ciprofloxacin and Macrobid. But these were prescriptions I got before pregnancy. Could I take them while pregnant? Was one better than the other? I huddled uncomfortably on the couch with my laptop, quickly locating a Web site that would tell me the FDA classifications of these drugs (www.safefetus.com). It seemed like Macrobid was a better bet, but the site said that there were "no adequate and well controlled studies done in humans" for *either* of the drugs. I finally broke down and paged my doctor, who assured me (sleepily) that taking Macrobid was fine.

The next morning, when I was feeling better and got a chance to look into it a bit more, I realized why my OB recommended one rather than the other. Macrobid is an FDA Category B drug, meaning that *although* there are no well-controlled studies in humans, animal studies have shown no risk to a fetus. In contrast, Cipro is a Category C drug. This means that there are also no studies in humans, and that *either* (1) studies in animals have shown problems for the fetus *or* (2) there have been no studies in animals.

When I looked a bit further, it seemed that basically everything was Category C in the United States (it turns out to be about 70 percent), meaning the FDA's attitude toward most drugs is equivocal. Further, the drugs that the FDA recommends avoiding aren't always the ones you'd expect. My intuition was that the stronger the drug, the more dangerous it would be for the fetus. But there are strong recommendations against taking Advil, and much less strong ones about Vicodin.

Of course, ideally you would never have to take any drugs during your pregnancy, but for most of us this is not realistic. For one thing, if you have something like a kidney infection, it's actually quite dangerous to leave it untreated. Even in cases where a drug might seem optional—back pain, chronic migraines, or even antidepressants—not taking medication can cause its own problems. Before making a choice one way or the other, it's important to understand a bit more about the possible downsides.

In thinking about this issue, I found it useful to start with some basic biology. Just like when I thought about the diet restrictions, having a general framework in which to think about drugs was more useful than thinking about each drug on its own. Without knowing about the biology, how was I supposed to start thinking about why one drug would be worse than another?

Your baby develops in your uterus and is connected to you through the placenta. The placenta is actually an incredibly unusual organ, which scientists are still working to fully understand. Among its neat properties is that it contains both Mom's and baby's blood and manages to keep them separate while at the same time transferring nutrients from Mom to baby and waste products from baby back out to Mom (for disposal).

Not too long ago doctors thought the placenta was an impenetrable barrier. It didn't matter what drugs or other substances pregnant women ingested, because nothing could affect the baby. One does wonder how, under this theory, the baby got any nourishment!

We now understand that this is very wrong. Pretty much whatever drug you are taking—over the counter, prescription, or illegal—the baby is getting exposed to it. Most drugs pass through by a process called *passive diffusion*, a fancy way of saying they just kind of soak through. If a drug doesn't get through the placenta, and therefore doesn't get to the baby, we can pretty much rule out the possibility that it's a problem. There are two types of drugs that either do not soak through or do so at only very minimal amounts: drugs that are too "large" and drugs that the placenta stores or processes.

Drugs with really big molecules do not pass through the placenta to the fetus. An example of this is heparin, a blood thinner. The heparin drug molecule is just so large and heavy that it literally cannot "fit" through the placenta. Think of the placenta as a sieve and heparin as a slightly-too-large piece of sand. This too-big issue can also happen with drugs that attach themselves to other substances, and through this process *become* too big to fit through. This is the case for glyburide, a drug commonly used to treat type 2 diabetes.[1] Sometime between ingestion and arrival at the placenta, glyburide links up with a large protein molecule and together they are too big to get through the placenta. Obviously, this is a very appealing feature of these drugs (at least as far as pregnancy is concerned): no transfer through the placenta, no direct effect on the baby.

The other reason why drugs might not get through is that some of them can get stuck in the placenta. For reasons that are really not understood, for a small number of drugs the placenta acts as a "depot." It just collects the drug and never passes it along. This is interesting, but probably not so relevant for most of the readers of this book. One of the most common drugs with this feature is buprenorphine, which is used to treat heroin withdrawal. If you do happen to be addicted to heroin, buprenorphine might be a better option than methadone. If not, it probably won't come up.

These categories are exceptions. In most cases—things like painkillers, antibiotics, or antidepressants—the baby consumes at least some of what you take. That *can* be a problem, but it isn't *necessarily* a problem. It really depends on the drug. That's where the FDA classification system comes in.

Drug Classes

Historically, the FDA splits the drugs pregnant women might take into five categories: A, B, C, D, and X. Category A drugs are the safest, and Category X drugs are the most dangerous. Although drugs will usually still report these classes, the FDA has started to require more detail about the reasoning behind these ratings, which is welcome.

Categories A, B, and C are all drugs for which there is no strong evidence of harm to human babies. The difference is in the quality of the evidence in people and the results of experiments in animals. Categories D and X are drugs that are contraindicated in pregnant women because studies have shown evidence of harm to babies from taking them. Category D includes drugs for which, although there is evidence of harm to babies, there *might* be a case for taking them, depending on the benefit to the mother. Class X drugs are those that absolutely should not be taken during pregnancy under any circumstances.

There isn't really as much information as I would have wanted about drugs. The FDA is equivocal about most drugs simply because it is hard to experiment on pregnant women (that's a good thing in general, just not for figuring out the dangers of drugs). Evidence from animals is useful, but goes only so far. Most of our data comes from nonexperimental evidence. Some women will take the drug because they have to or by accident, and researchers observe if there are any ill effects on the baby.

So, with the caveat that this is a case with tremendous uncertainty, let's take a look at these categories:

Category A: "Adequate, well-controlled studies in pregnant women have failed to demonstrate a risk to the fetus in any trimester of pregnancy."

It was almost impossible to find an example of a Category A drug. The FDA obviously has a very high (read: insane) standard for a well-controlled study. Most of the vitamins in my prenatal vitamins are not even Category A! The one example I could find was folic acid. The safety of folic acid has been supported in a large number of randomized studies of folic acid supplementation. But more than this, folic acid actually *prevents* birth defects. A review article published in 2010 summarized the evidence on this from randomized trials: women who took folic acid supplements were about 70 percent less likely to have a child with a neural tube birth defect (like spina bifida).[2] It may not only be birth defects: a large recent study in Norway suggested women who took folic acid before conception and during early pregnancy had children with much lower rates of autism.[3] In other words, this is not just safe, it's very highly recommended.

Not all Category A drugs necessarily have *benefits*, but if you do happen to come across one, you can be assured that it is very, very safe.

Category B: "Adequate, well-controlled studies in pregnant women have not shown increased risk of fetal abnormalities despite adverse findings in animals or, in the absence of adequate human studies, animal studies show no fetal risk."

Category B is slightly more common than Category A. A drug can be classified as B even without large randomized studies in humans as long as there are some good studies in humans or there is no risk shown in animals. Category B drugs typically have a lot of evidence in humans. For example, most of the things in your prenatal vitamins are Category B: many millions of women have taken them for years and there is no evidence of adverse effects. However, as there are no randomized trials (because randomly taking *away* prenatal vitamins would be unethical), these substances cannot technically be in the Category A bucket.

Other than prenatal vitamins, probably the most common Category B drug is **Tylenol** (or, more accurately, the active ingredient, **acetaminophen**). This is the most commonly used pain reliever during pregnancy; it seems likely that the majority of pregnant woman take it at some point.

Although there are no randomized trials in pregnant women, the evidence on the safety of Tylenol is vast, which is why it deserves the Category B ranking.[4] First, experimental studies in animals (mice and rats) show no impacts even at the rat equivalent of the maximum human dose. Second, there are large observational studies in humans that show no risk.

Among the biggest of these, one in Denmark followed more than 100,000 women. Half of these women reported taking acetaminophen at some time during pregnancy, and 30 percent did so in the first trimester (when doctors worry most about birth defects). The rates of birth defects among the exposed women were no higher than among those who didn't take the painkiller. This study also found no impact of exposure on miscarriage rate, stillbirth, or low birth weight.[5] There are a number of smaller studies that show similar results. The only demonstration of harm from Tylenol is among women who purposefully overdosed (and even this is hard to interpret, because most of these women simultaneously overdosed on something else).

With all of this evidence, it is not surprising that Tylenol has a favorable FDA rating; it's perhaps surprising that it is not the most favorable. In fact, in most other countries, acetaminophen is the equivalent of Category A. The United States classifications are significantly more stringent. As a result, few drugs even make it to Category B. Which brings us to the vast unwashed: Category C.

Category C: "Adequate, well-controlled studies in humans are lacking and animal studies have shown a risk to the fetus or there are not any animal studies. There is a chance of fetal harm if the drug is administered during pregnancy, but the potential benefits may outweigh the risk."

In layman's terms, drugs are characterized as Category C if there is no actual evidence of risk, but there is also no large-scale human data. This includes drugs where there is evidence of harm in animal studies, and those with no animal studies. It includes drugs with some small human studies, and those with no human studies.

One drug could have some small studies in people that show that things are fine, and also some nonrandomized studies in animals that show that things are fine. A second drug could have no human studies and animal studies that have shown fetal damage. And they'd both be in Category C! When I had my UTI, I couldn't figure out where Cipro fell in the Category C spectrum. It's an important difference: evidence of harm versus no evidence at all.

People smarter than me have noticed that Category C is less helpful than it might be, and there has been some push for the FDA to change this categorization. But for now, this is what we are stuck with. If your doctor wants to prescribe you a Category C drug, you have to push her on the evidence quality or look it up yourself.

One Category C drug frequently prescribed during pregnancy is **hydrocodone,** the active ingredient in both **Vicodin** and **Norco.** You'll probably get these prescribed if Tylenol isn't a significant enough painkiller.

Evidence on hydrocodone and pregnancy is limited. A search in medical abstracts for "Hydrocodone and pregnancy" yields eight results; a similar search for acetaminophen produces more than four hundred. Further, many of the existing studies are older and have small sample sizes. One of the few studies that comes up in a search is from 1996, and reports on just 118 women; this study finds no increased risk of birth defects among women exposed to hydrocodone.[6] Indeed, until recently this was probably the best evidence available on hydrocodone exposure in pregnant women.

Then, in early 2011, a new study was released that looked at this question in a much larger sample size (17,500 children with birth defects and 6,700 control children). The authors in this study found that using opioids in the first trimester of pregnancy was associated with an increased risk of heart defects and spina bifida. Their data set is still not large enough to single out hydrocodone relative to other drugs like it (codeine, for example). In addition, because these birth defects are not common, all the results are statistically weak.[7]

Nevertheless, this provides new evidence on the (possible) dangers of hydrocodone, evidence that will eventually be incorporated into the FDA classification system (my guess is that hydrocodone will stay Category C until more evidence comes in one way or the other). This is part of what is tricky about Category C: as the evidence evolves, drugs might seem more or less risky but remain in the same class. Given that you are pregnant now, and not sometime in the future, you'll have to make these decisions as best as you can with limited evidence.

And not everyone is going to make the same decision, even with the same evidence. When my sleepless friend, Heather, asked about Ambien (Category C) I sent her my evidence summary from the previous chapter—a couple of studies suggesting it was fine, and one small one indicating a risk of low birth weight from chronic use. I summarized: "This suggests to me it is fine to take occasionally." Heather disagreed—she argued that she was already worried about her son being small, and she didn't feel okay about it given the one discomforting study.

That, of course, is the value of evidence versus blanket rules. Rules assume everyone will make the same choice given the same evidence; showing people the evidence on their own allows them to make the choices that work for them.

Category D: "Studies in humans or investigational or postmarking data have demonstrated fetal risk. Nevertheless, potential benefits may outweigh the risk."

You really don't want to take a Category D drug unless you have to. These are drugs for which studies have shown some demonstrated risk to the fetus. Usually those risks are *relatively* minor; if something has a major risk it usually gets put in Category X. For Category D drugs, you and your doctor have to weigh the need for the drug against the risk of those relatively minor effects.

Consider an example: tetracycline, which is an antibiotic (in addition to the normal antibiotic uses, it also comes in handy in treating acne). Early on in the life of the drug, in 1964, an article in the *Journal of the American Medical Association* implicated tetracycline in tooth discoloration and possibly other bone issues.[8] This study is old, and it's *very* small: just 9 children. Having said this, 7 of the 9 children had tooth discoloration. Moreover, there is reason to think the drug might have this effect based on studies in adults.

This 9-person study is probably largely responsible for the Category D ranking. Once a drug falls into Category D (or worse, X), it will not be prescribed anymore, and it's therefore difficult to gather even observational data. The reason this drug is Category D and not Category X is that one can imagine a situation (say, this is the only available antibiotic) where you might want to prescribe the drug even with the risk of yellow teeth.

Category X: "Studies in animals or humans, or investigational or post-marking reports, have demonstrated positive evidence of fetal abnormalities or risk which clearly outweighs any potential benefit to the patient."

Category X drugs are strongly counterindicated during pregnancy. You shouldn't take them. The negative outcomes for the baby are serious, and likely, and the benefits of these drugs during pregnancy do not outweigh them.

The most commonly cited example is Accutane, which is a drug used to treat acute acne. It has been known more or less since the drug was introduced that it should not be taken during pregnancy. I think I was among the first wave of people to take Accutane, and I remember that the pills came in individual blister packs. On the back of *every pill* was a picture of a pregnant woman with an X marked through it. I believe they actually made me take a pregnancy test before prescribing this, despite the fact that I was twelve.

Still, there have been cases where pregnant women were accidentally exposed. A review article summarized the outcomes for

154 cases of accidental exposure.[9] Almost 100 women had elective abortions (either because the pregnancy was generally unplanned or due to the Accutane exposure). Of the remaining 59 pregnancies, 20 percent resulted in miscarriage and 35 percent had major birth defects. Both are much, much higher risks that you'd expect in the general population. And the birth defects were much more severe than tooth discoloration.

In addition, because Accutane is used almost exclusively to treat acne, it's difficult or impossible to imagine a situation where treatment of a skin condition would be more important than the health of the baby. Hence, Category X.

One caveat to keep in mind: drugs can also be Category X just because they have no purpose during pregnancy. Oral contraceptives are a Category X drug, but not because they are damaging to the baby.[10] This has relevance for a response to accidental exposure. After accidental exposure to Accutane, many women choose to terminate a pregnancy, knowing that the risk of life-threatening birth defects is very high. A similar response to accidental birth control pill exposure is not warranted. Although you should stop taking them after becoming pregnant (what's the point?), they are not implicated in birth defects.

It is pretty clear that any drugs in categories A and B are fine to take. Anything in categories D and X should be avoided unless truly necessary. The problem is Category C, where every drug is a little different in terms of the quality of the evidence. This leaves one with little choice but to try to read the actual evidence for every drug you might want to take. This is at best time consuming and at worst impossible. It would take the rest of this book (and be very boring!) to summarize the evidence on all popular drugs.

But armed with the knowledge about drug classifications, you can at least be a bit more informed when you ask your doctors about the drugs they prescribe. They should be able to evaluate the studies on risks, or at least point you in the right direction. In addition, in an appendix at the end of this book I provide a quick reference on drugs for a variety of common conditions. This way, if you wake up in the middle of the night with back pain or a migraine or an allergic reaction, you don't have to spend quite as much time on your laptop as I did!

A final note. Sometimes you actually *want* drugs to pass to the baby. An example is antiretrovirals for treating HIV. Researchers are working on ways to make this happen using molecules that actively transfer drugs across the placenta. In the long run, this could be used to treat diseases in fetuses before they are even born! At the moment, this is more in the realm of science fiction than reality, but it presents an exciting future.

The Bottom Line

- You should feel comfortable taking anything in pregnancy categories A and B.

- You should avoid anything in categories D and X (exceptions would be made for Category D drugs that treat very serious illnesses; this is doctor territory).

- For drugs in Category C, try to get a better idea of the safety evidence (either from your doctor or from the appendix here).

PART 4

The Third Trimester

. . .

Premature Birth (and the Dangers of Bed Rest)

There was a point in the middle of my pregnancy where I worried about the baby all the time. When I was at my parents' house for Christmas, around 22 or 23 weeks, there was a day in which I didn't feel Penelope move around at all. I'm told this is common—at that stage they are so small that if they get into an odd position you might not feel them—but it was hard not to freak out. I drank juice, I ate cookies. Nothing.

Because I'm generally a nervous person, at home we actually had a machine (called a Doppler) that you can use to hear the baby's heartbeat. It's a much cheaper version of what your doctor uses. I had already used it more than a few times in similar situations. But we were visiting my parents and hadn't brought it with us.

Not surprisingly, the Hamden, Connecticut, Walgreens doesn't stock a Doppler like this, so I bought a stethoscope. I quickly learned that it must take some training to be able to hear the baby with one of those—I had a hard time even picking up my own heartbeat.

In the end, Penelope was fine. Toward the end of the day she shifted position, and I experienced the reassurance of someone punching me as hard as she could in the bladder.

I had a few more days like this before Penelope was big enough that I could feel everything she did. Ultimately what I was afraid of was that something would happen in the womb and she would die (I find it difficult to write this, even now, knowing that she came out fine). This can happen, although, mercifully, it is rare. And, maybe paradoxically, for me this fear was made worse by knowing that by 25 or 26 weeks there is a better than 50 percent chance of survival outside the womb.

On the other hand, I was also worried about Penelope coming too early. Preterm birth (defined as before 37 weeks) is actually fairly common in the United States, occurring in about 12 percent of pregnancies. I didn't have any particular risk factors (no twins or triplets, for example), but I knew women who had unexpectedly gone into labor early without any warning signs.

In the end, as usual, I comforted myself with the numbers, and with information on what to do if I did go into labor too soon.

A premature birth is one that occurs between 22 and 36 weeks of pregnancy. The fact that this starts at 22 weeks is pretty incredible. As late as the 1960s, babies born even a few weeks premature frequently died. Among the most famous examples of this is John F. Kennedy's son, Patrick, who was born at about 34½ weeks, weighing almost 5 pounds, yet died two days later from respiratory disease. At the time, this wasn't a surprise. How things have changed: in 2005, 98.9 percent of babies born at that gestational age and weight survived their first year.[1]

Many of the advances in survival have been due to improvements in assisted ventilation. Lungs are among the last organs to develop (perhaps because they are not very useful when you are living in water), so babies born as late as 36 weeks can have serious trouble breathing. Mechanical breathing machines can be used until the baby is able to breathe on his own.

This and other advances have led to big improvements in survival for late-preterm infants (those born between 34 and 36 weeks) and also increases in the ability to save very, very preterm babies. At this point survival is possible (although not likely) at 22 or 23 weeks of gestation.

Prematurity, especially extreme prematurity, does have some long-term impacts. Babies born prematurely are more likely to get illnesses as children, on average have lower IQs, and often have vision or hearing problems. In one study of 5-year-olds born before 30 weeks of gestation, 75 percent of them had at least one disability (versus 27 percent among children born after 37 weeks). Their IQs were also 5 to 14 points lower, on average.[2] Moderate prematurity (32 to 36 weeks of gestation) also has had an impact on IQ in some studies, but these tend to be smaller and serious disabilities are less common.[3]

As I approached and passed 22, 23, and 25 weeks of pregnancy, the two key things I wanted to know were, first, what was the chance of having the baby each week? And second, if she did arrive early, what was the chance that she would survive? The Natality Detail Files provide information on every birth in the United States, including gestational week at birth as well as probability of death in the first year of life. The table on the next page has the answer (based on the 2005 data).

There are at least two very reassuring things about this data. First, although very preterm birth does happen, it's rare. Until 34 weeks, the chance of having a baby in any given week is less than 1 in 100. Before 30 weeks the chance in any given week is less than 1 in 500. Second, although survival rates are low for babies born early, they are not as low as you might have expected. More than half of babies born at 24 weeks will survive the first year— 24 weeks are just 5½ months pregnant. By the time you get to 28 weeks, still only 6½ months into pregnancy, the survival rate is almost 95 percent. These statistics have improved a lot even

Completed Weeks of Gestation	Percentage of Births	Probability of Death in the First Year
22	0.05%	77.1%
23	0.06%	62.6%
24	0.09%	39.3%
25	0.10%	26.0%
26	0.11%	18.1%
27	0.12%	13.6%
28	0.17%	7.5%
29	0.20%	5.5%
30	0.28%	4.0%
31	0.36%	3.2%
32	0.51%	2.1%
33	0.78%	1.5%
34	1.39%	1.1%
35	2.33%	0.8%
36	4.37%	0.6%
Full Term (37+)	89.09%	0.2%

since the early 1980s, when survival at 28 weeks was only about 80 percent.

Despite these fairly reassuring statistics, it's still better not to have your baby prematurely. There are some specific conditions that can prompt preterm labor (some of which are covered in the next chapter). Preterm labor can also occur for no apparent reason, and unfortunately modern medicine hasn't made a lot of progress on preventing it or stopping birth once it starts.[4] What doctors can do is give you one of a set of several tocolytic drugs (a common one is magnesium sulfate). These drugs will lessen contractions and can usually delay birth for a day or two (sometimes longer). What's the point in delaying just a couple of days? Two things: location and steroids.

A hugely important determinant of survival among very

preterm infants is the quality of care they receive and the types of interventions that are available to them. This, in turn, depends on the "level" of the NICU in the hospital in which you give birth. NICU levels range from 1 (which is basically just a nursery for healthy babies) to 4 (the highest level; in some states this is denoted 3C). The most advanced NICUs have the ability to do all types of neonatal surgery. They have ventilators and can often hook babies up to a heart-lung machine, which replicates the function of those two organs while they continue to develop.

Very premature babies are unlikely to survive without these interventions. Babies who are born very prematurely in hospitals without these capacities are typically transferred to more advanced hospitals once they are stable, but, if possible, it's better to be born in one of these in the first place. If birth can be delayed for a few days it is often possible to transfer Mom (while still pregnant) to a more advanced hospital. This means the baby will have the best possible care from the first moment.

In addition to location, the other intervention that makes a very large difference in survival is administering steroids. Steroid shots given to Mom speed up fetal lung development.[5] Even 24 hours of this treatment can make a huge difference: a recent review of randomized trials shows that steroids resulted in a 30 percent decrease in fetal death. Delaying birth for even a day or two lets doctors administer these drugs for long enough to make a difference.[6]

Babies are considered *early-term* at 37 weeks and *full-term* at 39 weeks of pregnancy. After 37 weeks most infants do not need any extra care after birth. Of course, the sharp distinction between preterm at 36-1/2 weeks and term at 37 weeks is artificial, and it is better for your baby to be born at 39 or 40 weeks rather than 37. But these differences are all small; infant mortality in the United States for nonpremature babies is just 2 in 1,000 births.

Bed Rest

In this discussion of preterm birth, steroid treatment, and NICU level, you may have noticed that bed rest didn't come up. On one hand, this is a bit of an omission on my part. Bed rest is very frequently prescribed for preterm labor. It's also common to prescribe it for a number of specific conditions—preeclampsia, for example, or cervical incompetence—that can lead to premature birth. Perhaps as many as 20 percent of women will be on bed rest for some of their pregnancy.

Bed rest is one of those solutions that is appealing, at least in part because it seems so logical. It seems as if you just lie down and stop jostling things around so much, that will help the baby stay inside. Also, if you know anyone who has been on bed rest, it probably looks like it worked out. Many women who are put on bed rest go on to have their babies at a normal time. But, and I cannot stress this enough, **that is not evidence that it works.** *You don't know what would have happened if those women had engaged in normal activities.*

In fact, there is no compelling evidence to suggest that bed rest is effective in preventing preterm labor.

There is a bit of randomized controlled trial evidence on this. In a study of 1,200 women with singleton pregnancies and threatened preterm labor, about 400 of them were put on bed rest and the other 800 were not. Bed rest was not effective at preventing preterm birth (7.9 percent of the bed rest group and 8.5 percent of the control group had their babies prematurely).[7] There's more randomized evidence for multiple gestations, and again, there is no evidence that women put on bed rest had fewer preterm deliveries or better general outcomes.[8]

There are also many, many review articles on this topic that look to other types of nonrandomized evidence. Nearly all suggest there is no evidence that this is effective. Here's a quote from one that was published in 2011: "There have been no complications of pregnancy for which the literature consistently demonstrates a benefit to ante-partum bed rest."[9] Here's another: "Research indicates, however, that bed-rest treatment is ineffective for preventing preterm birth and fetal growth restriction, and for increasing gestational age at birth and infant birth weight."[10] That last paper is actually titled "Lack of Evidence for Prescription of Antepartum Bed Rest."

Everyone agrees that more randomized evidence, with larger studies, would be better. But at the moment we simply have no evidence suggesting that bed rest works in improving outcomes for babies.

This wouldn't be such a big deal, except that bed rest actually has some significant negative consequences. Full bed rest is defined as one to two hours of activity per day, with the rest of the time spent in bed. No work, no running after your toddler, no setting up the baby's room, no making dinner, no exercise, no nothing. This has serious downsides for the rest of the family, and, for women who work, for their jobs. Studies cite financial strain on families when women are put on bed rest, even if they don't work, because of the need to get someone else to help around the house.

And even if you ignore these factors, there are actually medical risks to bed rest—bone loss, muscle atrophy, weight loss, and, in some studies, decreased infant birth weight.[11] There is some suggestion that it increases the risk of blood clots (to avoid this, women on bed rest sometimes wear compression socks).

Usually when we consider a medical treatment with no demonstrated benefits and large demonstrated risks, we think it's a bad idea. In fact, that's the strong consensus in the medical literature. And, even more surprising, many doctors seem to *know* this is a waste of time. A 2009 article that reported on a survey of practicing OBs shows that more than half of them said that bed rest has no or minimal benefit for any of these conditions.[12] And yet 90 percent of these doctors reported prescribing bed rest for some of these conditions. Even though they don't think it works!

What?

It would seem that this is one of those issues where the conventional recommendation has hung on despite evidence suggesting it's not just ineffective but damaging. There may be unusual situations in which bed rest is a good idea, but the medical literature hasn't found any of them. If your doctor suggests it you should almost certainly question her. Does she really think it will help despite all the evidence to the contrary?

The Bottom Line

- Survival outside the womb is possible (although not likely) as early as 22 weeks. Survival dramatically increases with continued gestation after this point. By 28 weeks, more than 90 percent of babies survive, and by 34 weeks it's 99 percent.

- Delaying birth after the onset of labor is difficult, but usually can be done for a few days. Delaying even just a day or two can have large impacts on survival by allowing you to be moved to a more advanced hospital, and giving time for steroid shots to improve the baby's lung function.

- There is no evidence that bed rest will prevent preterm labor. Avoid it.

High-Risk Pregnancy

W hen I hit 28 weeks of pregnancy, doctor appointments started coming every two weeks (and then, soon after, every week). For the most part, we were still pretty focused on discussing how fat I was getting (so fat!). But I also noticed around this time that the doctor was paying a bit more attention to how my belly was growing, listening more closely to the baby's heartbeat, and asking more probing questions about whether I was having any contractions.

There is a reason for this: it's often during the third trimester of pregnancy that problems start to emerge.

I will admit that I found the increase in doctor visits to be annoying. One problem was that my OB practice was always running late. I actually left one visit without even seeing the doctor after waiting an hour. I explained to them that I had to go, I had a meeting (which was true). They were really surprised—the receptionist kept telling me, "But everyone waits for the doctor!"

And some of the excess monitoring may have been unnecessary.

But for the most part even I, world's grumpiest patient, had to be very grateful for the improvements in medical technology in the past fifty, or even thirty, years. Doctors are better at detecting problems, and they are also better at fixing them. I had one pregnancy "issue": RH incompatibility. This is now so treatable that you might not even know you are being treated for it (just another of many shots). But as late as 1960 this was a major source of infant anemia, heart failure, and death.

There is still a ways to go in a lot of these pregnancy problems, but progress has been made, and continues.

If you end up with a high-risk-pregnancy condition, your doctor is going to be your best resource. The treatments tend to be very specific to the individual—to your case and the particular details of your baby. For this reason I wondered whether this information even belonged in this book. I don't have any special expertise on this subject. All I have is an introductory obstetrics textbook and some friendly doctors to whom I ask questions.[1]

But then my friends started popping up with these conditions here and there, and began asking me about them. I realized that in a lot of cases these problems were diagnosed and people weren't told the first thing about them. At 32 weeks my friend Daphna was told: "Your baby looks a little small. It's not something to worry about, but we'll start doing ultrasounds every week to see what is going on."

Perhaps my friends and I are a bit obsessive. But surely if something necessitates ultrasounds every week, it is, in fact, something to worry about. Or, at the very least, something to find out more about. After the conversation with her doctor Daphna spent hours on the computer, trying to figure out the long-term consequences of intrauterine growth restriction. Was she worried? Well, frankly, yes.

It's hard to accept a faceless diagnosis and a standard treatment without knowing just a bit more about what is going on and how worried you should be. The chart below is far from complete; it's just a starting point. As you might expect, one of the commonly suggested treatments for a number of these conditions is bed rest. Same story as the previous chapter: question and avoid.

Will It Happen Again?

With all these complications, if they do happen in a first pregnancy, a natural question is whether they are likely to happen again in later pregnancies. Unfortunately, the answer is generally yes. This is true for two reasons. First, there are some observable characteristics of people that relate to their risks. Overweight women, for example, are at higher risk for many of these complications (gestational diabetes, hypertension). If you are overweight with one pregnancy, you are likely to be overweight with another.

But beyond this, it would seem that these risks are linked to some genetic or physiological feature of particular women. This means that if you have a complication once, it is an indication that you are the type of woman who is at higher risk for that complication. In some cases, like with cervical insufficiency, it's a virtual certainty: if you have this with one baby, you'll have it with the next. In others, like preeclampsia, your risk is increased if it has happened before, but it is by no means a certainty.

PLACENTA PREVIA

Placenta partially or fully covers the cervix

Possible consequences

- Vaginal bleeding with potential for significant blood loss
- Preterm birth

Possible management/treatments

- Need for Cesarean delivery
- Vast majority resolve on their own
- Follow-up ultrasound after initial diagnosis to confirm
- If condition continues to term, Cesarean delivery typically around 36–37 weeks

PLACENTAL ABRUPTION

Placenta detaches, partially or fully, from the wall of the uterus

Possible consequences

- Painful contractions and vaginal bleeding with potential for significant blood loss
- Preterm birth
- Fetal growth restriction
- Need for Cesarean delivery

Possible management/treatments

- If full term, treatment is delivery
- If preterm, management varies with degree of abruption
- If there is concern about the fetal or maternal condition, delivery may be indicated even if the baby is preterm

GESTATIONAL DIABETES

Diabetes diagnosed during pregnancy

continued

Possible Consequences

- Possibility of a very large baby, which leads to:

    Obstetric risks—need for instruments or C-section

    Fetal/neonatal risks—stillbirth, shoulder stuck in delivery, metabolic problems

Possible managment/treatment

- Glucose monitoring and control through diet and exercise modification, or with medications if needed

RH ALLOIMMUNIZATION

Baby has positive blood type, Mom has negative

Possible Consequences

- If the maternal body is exposed to the fetus's Rh(D)-positive red blood cells, antibodies are produced that can cross the placenta and flag the fetus's red blood cells for destruction

- Can result in severe fetal and neonatal anemia and hyperbilirubinemia

Possible managment/treatment

- Rhogam shot given at 28 weeks and after delivery—a simple triumph of modern medicine

CERVICAL INSUFFICIENCY

Painless dilation of the cervix

Possible Consequences

- Can cause second trimester miscarriage or very preterm birth

continued

Possible managment/treatment

- Cervical length screening, progesterone treatment, or need for a cerclage—putting a stitch in the cervix to keep it closed

FETAL GROWTH RESTRICTION

A fetus that is small and not reaching its growth potential. Risk factors may include smoking, malnutrition, placental problems, or intrinsic fetal problems.

Possible Consequences

- Very low birth weight, preterm birth, stillbirth or neonatal death, metabolic and breathing problems

Possible managment/treatment

- Continual evaluation of fetal growth, behavior, amniotic fluid, and blood flow in fetal vessels
- May need early delivery when the baby would be better off outside the womb than inside

PREECLAMPSIA, ECLAMPSIA, HELLP SYNDROME

Related disorders that involve high blood pressure, with an increased amount of protein in the urine. Occurs after 20 weeks of pregnancy. Possible symptoms may include headache, visual disturbances, abdominal pain, and sudden weight gain.

Possible Consequences

- Eclampsia is a complication of preeclampsia that involves seizures
- HELLP is a complication that results in hemolysis (destruction of red blood cells), elevated liver enzymes (liver dysfunction), and low platelets
- Death of mother or baby if not treated

continued

Possible managment/treatment

- Evaluation includes assessment of blood pressure, blood tests, urine collection for protein measurement, and how well the baby is doing and growing
- Magnesium sulfate +/- blood pressure medications are used to prevent seizure or stroke
- Treatment is delivery of baby and placenta
- Delivery preterm may be needed in severe cases

PLACENTA ACCRETA

Abnormal invasion of the placenta into the wall of the uterus. There is increased risk of having this if you have placenta previa or have had prior Cesarean deliveries.

Possible Consequences

- Massive hemorrhage at the time of delivery, especially if not diagnosed prior to delivery

Possible managment/treatment

- Delivery by Cesarean section, immediately followed by hysterectomy

Notes for this table: 2, 3, 4, 5, 6, 7, 8, 9, 10, 11, 12, 13

I'm Going to Be Pregnant Forever, Right?

A t some point you blessedly stop worrying about having a premature baby. Almost immediately you switch to the opposite concern: that the baby will never arrive.

My mother told me that the end of pregnancy is so uncomfortable so that you'll be less afraid of labor. I'm not sure if there is a good scientific reason behind this argument, but she's right. By 37 or 38 weeks I got more uncomfortable every day. By the end it was all I could do to waddle downstairs in the morning, get my cup of coffee, and go watch TV. When I did go into work people would stop by my office to look at me with pity and ask, "No baby yet?"

It's around this point that many women become convinced they will be pregnant "forever." This intensifies as the due date comes and goes. In fact, without intervention most women (especially with their first baby) will still be pregnant when 40 weeks rolls around. According to at least one study, without any intervention, the average woman pregnant with her first child goes into labor a full *8 days* after her supposed "due date."[1] The good news is that you will not be pregnant forever. Even without medical induction (which is virtually certain to happen by 42 weeks), the baby is coming out eventually.*

I was actually pretty curious about when this "eventually" was. Jesse was scheduled to teach pretty much right up to my due date. At some point he asked whether he needed to put someone on notice to teach his class, and if so, for how many weeks? What was the chance of labor in the thirty-eighth week?

If you're wondering about this from the vantage point of early pregnancy, as we were, what you want to know is what share of babies are born by week. I sent Jesse the following chart, which shows the share of women (only those with singleton pregnancies— no twins, who tend to come earlier) delivering their baby by week of pregnancy. This is based on *all* births in the United States in 2008 (the last year of available data), so it is pretty precise.[2]

You are most likely to have your baby in your 39th week of pregnancy: close to 30 percent of babies are born in this week. The next most common week is week 38 (18 percent), followed by the 40th week (17 percent). About 70 percent of babies are born before their due date. This includes all births; first births and those that are not induced tend to be a bit later.

I think this chart got passed around more than any of the other data I produced during pregnancy. Everyone wanted to plan around something. In our case, Jesse did enlist a colleague to be on standby for his class, but it was unnecessary. Penelope waited until two days after her dad's grades were in to make an appearance.

As I got toward the end of pregnancy, though, this wasn't quite the right picture. If you get to your due date with no baby, it's hardly useful to know that you had a 70 percent chance of

---

* In 1945, *Time* magazine reported on a woman who claimed to have been pregnant for 53 weeks prior to giving birth to a 6 pound 15 ounce baby. It seems likely, however, that this woman suffered a miscarriage and then reconceived. Given that her husband was fighting in World War II at the time, one can imagine how a 53-week pregnancy might have been convenient.

Share of Births by Week of Gestation

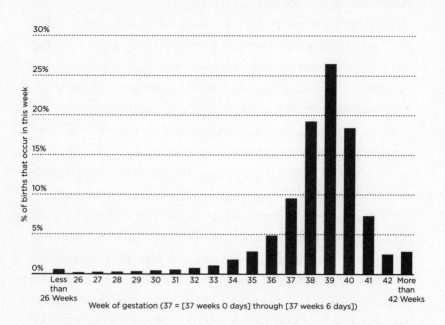

Week of gestation (37 = [37 weeks 0 days] through [37 weeks 6 days])

already having the baby. Obviously that didn't happen! A better way to ask the question: Sitting there, still pregnant, at the start of week 38, what's the chance that you'll be a mom by the beginning of week 39? It turns out that the same data, a bit reorganized, can tell you that, as well.

Week of pregnancy	Chance of birth this week if still pregnant at start of week
35th week	3%
36th week	5%
37th week	11%
38th week	25%
39th week	46%
40th week (first week **after** due date)	59%
41st week	58%
42nd week (including induction)	virtually 100%

If you get to your due date without a baby, there is a 60 percent chance you'll have the baby in the next 7 days. If you haven't had the baby by 41 weeks, there is about a 60 percent chance you'll go into labor spontaneously. At 42 weeks the vast majority of doctors will induce labor.

This is just an average. Around this time, the doctor visits ramp up to at least once a week—sometimes twice a week. My doctor, at least, also started in with the cervical checks. The idea behind these checks is to give a sense of whether you are progressing toward labor. Normally, your cervix is closed. In the time leading up to labor and, mostly, during labor, the cervix opens to 10 centimeters.

It also undergoes other changes—it *softens* and *shortens* and *thins*. At the same time, the baby moves down in your pelvis. This movement of the baby (*dropping*, or *lightening*) usually occurs a few days or weeks (or a couple of months, even) prior to labor (it can also occur during labor). For some people, the opening, softening, and thinning of the cervix also starts to occur in the days or weeks before labor starts.

This is what the doctor is looking for at the cervical checks. They'll report any progress—something like, "You are already one centimeter dilated!" You might think that this is a good sign that you'll be going into labor soon. After all, these cervical checks are painful, so you'd hope there is some information being gained.

The state of the cervix does have some predictive power, especially on or after your due date. But if you are expecting some kind of crystal ball, think again. Plenty of women go into labor without any sign at their cervical checks. On the flip side, my sister-in-law walked around for weeks with her second child while she was 3 centimeters dilated. They kept telling her, "This weekend!" Not very helpful, but also not that unusual.

In practice, although your doctor is more likely to tell you about dilation, cervical length (*effacement*) is probably a better predictor of labor onset.[3] Your doctor is measuring this at the same time that she is measuring whether you are dilated, so it's reasonable to ask her about it if she is doing a cervical check. It's usually reported as a percent ("You are 50 percent effaced," for example), which captures how far you have gone between the normal nonpregnant situation (0 percent effaced) and what will happen at delivery (100 percent effaced).

The most precise data I could find on this comes from one study in the United Kingdom that measured this effacement by ultrasound at 37 weeks, and then recorded the chance of going into labor by the due date.[4] The graph below shows their results. For women who were more than 60 percent effaced (that means shortened about halfway) at 37 weeks, almost all of them (something like 98 percent) went into labor before their due date. On

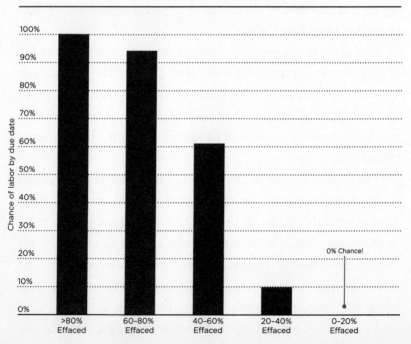

Cervical Length and Labor Timing

the other hand, for women who were less than 40 percent effaced, almost none of them (less than 10 percent) went into labor before their due date.

You may decide (some women do) that you want to skip the cervical checks. Some people figure that the baby is eventually coming out one way or another, so how valuable is this information, anyway? But it can be pretty useful. When my friend Heather was expecting her second baby, her plan was to fly her mother in to take care of baby number one while she and her husband were at the hospital.

At 37 weeks she was 1 centimeter dilated and 80 percent effaced. She took a look at this graph, and moved her mother's flight up by ten days. Not a moment too soon: her mother arrived on a Thursday afternoon, and baby boy followed on Saturday night. Evidence in action!

In addition to cervical length on its own, there is a more comprehensive measure of how far you have progressed, called the Bishop score. This is a number (between 0 and 13) that takes into account various things about the cervix (its position, how effaced you are, how dilated you are) and the position of the baby (very high up, or low down). A high Bishop score implies that you are further along. It also indicates an increased chance of a vaginal delivery; usually a score of 6 or above is seen as fairly advanced.

In terms of time to labor, it's not clear that this is much better than just knowing the effacement number, but some studies have shown that combining the two is especially helpful.[5] If you are curious, your doctor should be able to tell you this score when he does the cervical check.

You might wonder: if these measures are good at predicting onset of labor after you reach full term, maybe they could also be used to predict (and prevent) premature babies? In practice, both cervical length and the overall Bishop score do predict preterm labor,[6] but the predictive power is much weaker. Unless you are at risk for premature delivery (i.e., you're pregnant with twins, or you've had a premature baby before), you are unlikely to have your cervix checked before your thirty-seventh week, so it is probably a moot point.

A final note. Both the Bishop score and cervical length alone are very predictive of the outcome of induced labor: the more ready you are, the more likely the induction will lead to a vaginal delivery (versus a C-section).[7] This is another reason to pay attention to them. If you do end up considering a medical induction but you want to avoid a C-section, they can give you a good sense of the risks.

The Bottom Line

- No one has ever been pregnant forever.

- The majority of babies arrive within a week on either side of your due date.

- Cervical checks are predictive of coming labor (although not perfectly); ask about effacement in addition to dilation to get a more complete picture.

Labor Induction

My OB started talking about labor induction around 39 weeks of pregnancy. She wasn't pushy about it, but she wanted to start a dialogue about when we would schedule it. A few days after the due date?

I told her I wasn't interested, and that was it for the moment. She said we could revisit it when I was a few days overdue (Penelope had fortunately arrived by then). In fact, my OB practice was fairly lenient on this; they told me they'd let me go to 42 weeks, as long as the baby seemed to be doing okay. Other friends at other practices had their doctors pushing induction starting at the due date, and insisting on it at 41 weeks.

Medical induction is increasingly routine, but it wasn't always like this. Not that long ago, doctors were actually somewhat reluctant to induce labor until quite late. In 1990 (the first year in which this is recorded in the national data), fewer than 10 percent of births followed medical induction of labor. By 2008 the number had grown to 25 percent. Inductions done before the due date have actually changed the length of pregnancy in the United States. In 1980, 55 percent of births occurred on or after the stated due date, and by 2008 this figure had dropped to just 33 percent.

There are two ways that induction can be done. If your cervix is starting to soften and dilate on its own, induction is done with Pitocin, a synthetic version of the natural hormone oxytocin, which starts contractions. If your cervix is not ready on its own, doctors will often start with a prostaglandin drug (misoprostol is an example) or an apparatus called a *balloon catheter*. The drug softens the cervix; the balloon just stretches it out. These are likely to be combined with Pitocin. The advantage of either (over Pitocin alone) is that the induction is less likely to lead to a C-section.[1]

Regardless of how you do it, medical induction is very likely to be successful in the sense that after it is done, you have a baby.

What my doctor was offering me was, in essence, an elective induction. I could choose to have the baby at 40 weeks rather than wait for her to arrive on her own. And by 39 weeks I was definitely tired of being pregnant and Penelope was plenty big.

And yet I wanted nothing to do with this. There were basically two reasons.

First, use of Pitocin may increase pain in labor. For anecdotal evidence on this all you have to do is go to the Internet: chat boards are full of women who have had both spontaneous labor and an induction and report that the latter was more unpleasant. My mother had three children, all without an epidural, and reported that the labor she had with my youngest brother after she was induced was the worst, despite the fact that he was the third kid. Going beyond anecdotes, researchers find that women who are induced with Pitocin are more likely to use an epidural; increased use of pain relief probably points to increased pain (at least before the epidural was administered!).[2]

Second, there is some evidence that induction can increase the risk of a C-section, mostly when Pitocin is used alone.[3] Of course,

C-sections are safe and common, but recovery from them still tends to be harder than recovery from a vaginal delivery.

These concerns are there for any induction—before or after 40 weeks. I was even more wary of pre-due-date induction. Some women like this idea—37 weeks is full term, so why not get the baby out already?—but it is really not a good idea.

It is true that babies who come out on their own at 37 weeks do pretty much just as well as those who arrive on their own at 40 weeks (one measure of this is the percentage of babies with low APGAR scores: 9 in 1,000 at 37 weeks and 8 in 1,000 at 40 weeks). But this is only among babies who arrive on their own. Among induced births, those at 37 weeks do *worse* than those at 40.

Some babies are ready at 37 weeks, but that does not mean they all are. Recognizing this, in 2014 the American Congress of Obstetricians and Gynecologists reclassified 37 to 38 weeks of pregnancy as "early term" rather than "full term" and argued that inductions in this period should only be done if medically necessary.

As is typical for me, as soon as I realized I didn't *want* an induction, I got paranoid that it would be forced on me. This could happen for one of a few reasons:

1. Most doctors, even pretty permissive ones, don't like to let patients go past 42 weeks.

2. Your water breaks before contractions start (despite what you see on TV, this happens for only about 10 percent of women).

3. Your health is declining: preeclampsia, hypertension, gestational diabetes.

4. The baby is not "tolerating" continued pregnancy: low fluid readings or failure on a non-stress test.

I realized pretty quickly that in the first three cases there wasn't much I could do to prevent an induction, and probably not much I wanted to do. Although some people will argue with this (people will argue with anything), there is reasonable evidence that staying pregnant past 42 weeks is risky for the baby.[4] If your water breaks, labor will often start on its own, but if it doesn't, induction limits the risk of an infection to the baby (more on this later). And, of course, if your own health is at risk, that is a very good reason to induce.

But the last one worried me. Increasingly, inductions are done because of a worry that the baby isn't tolerating pregnancy well. There are two main monitoring technologies doctors use for this: amniotic fluid levels, and something called a *non-stress test*.

There are good reasons to use these. Knowing more about how the baby is doing inside the womb can literally save lives. For the high-risk pregnancy conditions I talked about a few chapters ago, continual monitoring is extremely helpful and we are lucky to have it.

Having said this, these tests are, at best, pretty coarse. Especially for low-risk women with normally developing pregnancies, they sometimes seem to cause more harm than good.

Once I got into my anti-induction paranoia, I kept hearing about people who were induced after these tests. The fluid seemed to be the biggest issue: at least three friends pregnant within a year of me were induced due to low amniotic fluid. And in all these cases the whole thing came as a surprise. They went for a routine visit, and all of a sudden were told they needed an induction right away, with no time for processing what had gone on or thinking about whether it was the right decision.

It is not that I wanted to avoid the tests. Economics teaches a basic view that more information is better than less. But I wanted to make sure I understood them well enough that I didn't fail them for the wrong reason.

Monitoring of Amniotic Fluid

Inside your uterus your baby swims around in a large pool of amniotic fluid. If the pool gets too low, you can develop a condition called *oligohydraminos* (catchy!), which just means low amniotic fluid. The danger is that if the fluid level gets too low, the umbilical cord can get compressed. Think about it like a pool: as the water gets lower, you are more likely to be pressed up against the side rather than floating. If the cord is caught between the baby and the side of the uterus, it's harder for blood to flow through it. Low fluid can also indicate that the placenta isn't doing its job correctly, which could point to other problems.

This is a real and significant concern. Babies born to mothers with consistently low fluid readings are more likely to need time in the NICU, and their mortality rates are higher.[5] Low fluid can also be a marker for other problems, like fetal growth restriction. If you have a low fluid reading there is good reason to do other tests (like the non-stress test described below) to make sure nothing else is going on with the baby. If there are other signs that the baby is not doing well, especially at full term, inducing labor is generally recommended.

But not all low fluid readings indicate a problem. Low fluid in the absence of any other problem is called *isolated oligohydraminos*. This would be a case where everything else about the baby looks normal—good size on the ultrasound; moving well in a non-stress test—and the only issue is a low fluid level. It is common for doctors to induce labor in this case, especially if you are full term or close to full term.[6] This is what happened with my various friends—low fluid at term equals induction.

And yet despite this common practice there is little evidence suggesting that these isolated low-fluid readings warrant induction.[7] To the extent that there *is* evidence, it suggests that babies do as well with "expectant management" (jargon for leaving you alone). One small (54 women) randomized study compared women induced for an isolated low-fluid reading versus those who were not induced and found no difference in what happened with their babies.[8] A second study randomized women into screening for this issue, and then tracked the growth of their babies. They found that increased screening did identify more cases of this, but babies with isolated low-fluid readings were no different in terms of growth and outcome than those who had normal fluid.[9]

Yet a third article, this one about detection of this issue before 37 weeks of pregnancy, argued that babies with this condition did worse *but mostly because the mothers were induced early!* When the authors limited to women who were diagnosed with *oligohydraminos* but chose not to induce, their babies looked quite similar to those with normal fluid levels.[10]

Knowing all this did nothing to stem my paranoia. I was now *convinced* this was a bad idea, but worried that I wouldn't be able to do anything about it. One couple I know ended up inducing in this situation even though the father was a doctor and a medical researcher, and aware of the literature. The pressure from the doctor was just too strong.

I am always up for a fight (especially with evidence on my side!), but it seemed like the best option was to avoid having low fluid in the first place. It turns out there are a few ways to do this.

The first is to make sure your doctor is measuring the fluid in the most reliable way. Fluid levels are measured on an ultrasound. The ultrasound tech takes a few measurements and uses them to calculate how much fluid there is. They can report the amount of fluid in two ways: total fluid volume (also called AFI) or the depth of the "deepest vertical pocket."

Once again, imagine your uterus as a pool, this time with a deep end and a shallow end. The total fluid volume measures the amount of water in the pool; the deepest vertical pocket measures the depth of water in the deepest part of the deep end.

As measurements go, the deepest-vertical-pocket measure is much better. It captures the same number of truly problematic situations but is much better at *not* identifying cases where there is nothing wrong.[11] It leads to fewer inductions and fewer C-sections. It's easy to see why: your baby has a choice of where to hang out in the uterus, so as long as there is an area of the deep end of the pool with enough water, it's really not that important how high the water is in the shallow end. Although it is more common to use the total amount of fluid, it makes sense to push them to take both measurements.

The second solution, even easier, is hydration. In several randomized trials it has been shown that having women drink two liters of water before their ultrasound dramatically increases their fluid levels.[12] This is a lot of water, and you're really going to have to pee afterward, but it's not a complicated intervention!

Finally, if your readings are borderline, you may want to push for a repeat measurement rather than agreeing to an immediate induction. When my friend Jane went in on her due date, she had a borderline low reading, followed by another one the next day. The doctor scheduled an induction, but Jane pushed for one more measurement the day before the induction—at which point the level was higher, so they canceled the induction and let her go another week. By this time we joked that perhaps she shouldn't have listened to me. But in the end she was glad to have waited, especially because her son was on the smaller side.

Non-Stress Test

Despite my fears, or perhaps because of them, I passed the fluid test with no incident on my due date. I had forced Jesse to come with me to the doctor, just in case we had to fight (with the OB, not with each other). After the fluid, I told him he could leave.

"Are you sure?" he asked. I told him to go. There was a second test, but I didn't know anyone who had failed it, so I wasn't worried.

After he was gone, they took me to an exam room and hooked up the non-stress test. It's pretty simple: they put you on a fetal monitor for an extended period of time (usually about twenty minutes). The intent is to make sure the baby is still moving around and doing his thing in there.

This is basically just a fancier version of the system from our mothers' generation where they had women count their baby's movements. The NST continually measures the fetal heart rate. Babies who are moving around should show variation over time in their heart rate. It's similar to how this would work in adults. If you are just lying around, your heart rate is fairly constant; when you start to move around, it accelerates. When doctors look at the NST, they look for these heart-rate accelerations to indicate that the baby is active.

The only problem with this test is that it doesn't work great (or really at all) when the baby is asleep. Which is actually quite a lot of the time. About 30 percent of NSTs are what is called *nonreactive*, which means that although you can hear the heartbeat fine, it's not changing much.

If your baby fails this test, it could be that she is sleeping (which would be fine) or that she is in trouble (which would not be fine). One simple way to increase the precision of these tests is to do them at night, when babies are more likely to be awake (as you presumably know from waking up at four A.M. to find that your baby is having a uterus party). But most doctors don't schedule four A.M. visits.

Given that such a large percentage of babies fail these tests due to sleeping, doctors will usually do a number of things to try to wake up the baby before they start to worry. Among the most effective of these interventions is a very simple one: clapping.[13] In one study, 485 women were given these tests and initially 143 of them failed. For these women, the researcher then clapped loudly 3 to 5 times right on top of the abdomen. This got the attention of most babies: 92 percent of the babies who were previously asleep had a normal test result after the clapping.

Many doctors will also suggest sugar. Tasty, but evidence suggests it is completely ineffective.[14] Clapping is a better bet.

You can also take your own approach. Despite my assurances to Jesse, Penelope wasn't doing so well on movement when we were first hooked up. They left me there for 10 minutes, 20 minutes, then 30 minutes. Occasionally someone would come in, look at the monitor, and make some concerned noise.

I knew we weren't doing so well, so I took it up with Penelope. I had a long talk with her and indicated that if she didn't wake up she was going to fail her very first test. The threat of failure is a real motivation for Oster women: she woke up immediately. Of course, clapping might have been easier, and perhaps less psychologically damaging.

A final note: if your baby doesn't respond to clapping and other attempts to wake him up, it is definitely time to take action. Truly nonreactive NSTs are often associated with fetal distress. In the clapping study, of the 11 women who didn't respond to clapping, 5 of them responded after being given oxygen. But of the remaining 6 truly nonresponsive babies, half of them really *were* in distress and would have been in trouble without an emergency C-section.

The Bottom Line

- Best option: go into labor on your own.

- Prebirth fetal monitoring is a good idea, but beware of false positives.

- Fluid monitoring. Two easy ways to avoid false positives: (1) stay hydrated, and (2) ask your doctor to measure the deepest vertical pocket rather than total fluid volume.

- Non-stress test. Advice: just keep clapping.

Do-It-Yourself "Induction"

Somewhere between the extremes of doing nothing and medical induction lies the realm of natural, do-it-yourself induction methods. The Internet is full of these—women suggest everything from herbs to walking to sex. One reason women try these is, of course, that they are tired of being pregnant. But they also have the potential to avoid a medical induction. As the due date comes and goes, some women, like me, start to worry that their doctor will want to induce, and they'd like to try something—anything—to have labor come on its own.

The methods here shouldn't really be called induction in the sense that they don't necessarily lead to labor. They're more like "labor encouragement." Actually, for the most part there is no evidence that they even do that. On the other hand, there is no real evidence of harm from them, and if it makes you feel better to do something, go for it. Here's a quick rundown of the main chat-board options.*

Red Raspberry Leaf Tea: There is not much theory on this one, except that people have been using it for a long time. There might be a temptation to be convinced by this alone—midwives have been recommending it for hundreds of years!—but the truth is that because everyone eventually goes into labor, anything that you recommend women to take is going to look like it works some of the time.

What evidence there is on this doesn't suggest much impact on the timing of labor onset.[15] At least one study evaluated its role in shortening labor, and also found no impact.[16] It's unlikely to hurt you to have a nice cup of tea, but if that's what you want, you might just as well have some English Breakfast.

Evening Primrose Oil: This has the distinction of being something one of the OBs in my practice actually recommended—at least, she said I should consider it if I wasn't dilated at all by 37 weeks. The idea is that you either take this oil in a pill form or use it as a vaginal suppository. Despite the doctor-approved stamp, this isn't actually supported by evidence. In fact, one small study showed it had no impact on the length of labor and actually *increased* the risk of both your water breaking early and needing instruments to help get the baby out.[17]

Sex: Most women are not feeling their sexiest at 40 weeks pregnant. But if sex is what it takes to get things moving, maybe that will help get you in the mood. In fact, the idea that sex might trigger labor does have some science behind it: semen contains a chemical that prompts cervical dilation.

In practice, although there is more evidence on this than there is on the various herbs, it is largely inconclusive. In nonrandomized

---

* There are some things left out here, like eggplant and spicy food and waving a charcoal stick above your belly (really!). Some people will try anything! There's no real evidence on these other methods one way or the other.

studies, people who had sex late in pregnancy were less likely to need medical induction of labor.[18] However, at least one randomized study suggested there was no impact. You might wonder how you randomize sex. The researchers randomly *encouraged* some couples to have sex and did not encourage others (they didn't discourage them; they just didn't say anything one way or the other). More couples who were encouraged to have sex did so (60 percent, versus 40 percent in the control), but there was no noticeable effect on going into labor. Again, it's not going to kill you to do it, but it's also probably not going to move things along.[19]

Acupuncture: The morning of my due date, on the advice of our doula, I scheduled an acupuncture session for the next day (what can I say? I was impatient!). Then later that day I went into labor. Even the threat of acupuncture worked! I feel a bit bad that I never called to cancel the appointment, but I *was* pretty busy.

I was compelled to try this method by my trust in our doula, but also by a 2009 review article that described two randomized studies suggesting that acupuncture is effective in promoting labor. Although both studies had small sample sizes, together they suggested that women with acupuncture are about 1.5 times as likely to go into labor on their own.[20] Sounded good to me.

As it happens, more recent studies have questioned this conclusion. One trial compared labor-inducing acupuncture to "sham" acupuncture (i.e., done at the wrong points on the body) and concluded that a similar percentage of women went into labor after two treatments.[21] A slightly larger study (also randomized) confirmed this "no effect" conclusion.[22]

Nipple Stimulation: Finally, something that might actually work. Breast stimulation causes your uterus to contract, and there is evidence that this can induce labor. A review article reported on four studies that randomized full-term pregnant women into a "breast stimulation" or "no breast stimulation" group and recorded whether they had gone into labor 3 days later.[23]

Of the breast stimulation group, 37 percent were in labor by 3 days, versus only 6 percent of those without breast stimulation! This is a large effect, and was very consistent across all studies. There was also some reduction in the risk of postpartum hemorrhage, a significant postbirth complication.

It sounds great: no needles, you can do it at home, it has other benefits, and it works to induce labor! The only downside is that it is awfully time consuming. The women in these studies were asked to massage their breasts for at least an hour a day for 3 days; in two cases, it was an hour *3 times a day*. That's a lot of time. In some cases the women used a breast pump. Less work, still a lot of time. On the other hand, for me at least, the last few days of pregnancy were spent mostly on the couch watching television. Perhaps I could have put the time to better use.

Membrane Stripping/Sweeping: Technically, membrane stripping is not something you can do on your own. I've put it in the natural-labor-induction category, however, because, unlike other medical induction of labor, it's intended to increase the chance of going into labor spontaneously.

The procedure for doing this is very simple, and can be done by your doctor while performing a cervical check. During the exam, the doctor puts her finger through the cervix and detaches the membranes (the bag of water holding the baby) from the wall of the uterus. It's called *sweeping* because it's done by sweeping the finger around in a circle.

And it works. It's typically done at or after your due date. Women who had this done were more likely (about 25 percent more) to go into labor within 2 days. They were less likely to still be pregnant at 41 or 42 weeks. This procedure even works on women whose cervices are unfavorable (meaning not dilated or effaced much), which makes them less likely to go into labor on their own without it.[24] There don't seem to be many downsides—no increase in C-section, for example, and similar outcomes for the babies (the only downside identified is that this procedure is painful for most women).

The Bottom Line

- Tea, oil, sex—all duds at starting labor.

- Acupuncture evidence is mixed.

- Nipple stimulation works, and so does membrane stripping (but don't do this last one at home).

PART 5

Labor and Delivery

. . .

The Labor Numbers

Compared to the total pregnancy, labor is quite short. Yet it occupies an outsize percentage of attention. You can see why, of course. Labor is definitely the most "medical" part of pregnancy, it involves a huge number of decisions (by you, and also possibly by your doctor), and it's, frankly, a little scary.

Most people have some rough idea of how labor works. If you don't, you'll get it at even the barest-bones prenatal class. Jesse and I went to just one day of labor "prep" at the hospital where I had Penelope. The summary of labor was along the lines of: first the baby is inside, then you go into labor, the cervix opens, and then later the baby is outside. Ta da! There was also a visual demonstration involving a doll and a turtleneck.

This description is, of course, basically correct. You may feel like it is enough. One couple in our prenatal class was more concerned with whether they could get their child's footprints put directly into their baby book than with the details of what occurred between "the baby is inside" and "the baby is outside." But, as usual, I wanted more details.

Labor occurs in three stages. At the start, your baby is still in

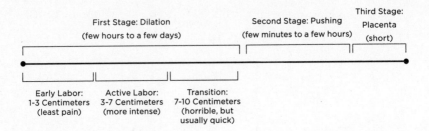

the uterus, and the cervix at the bottom is closed. By the end, both the baby and the placenta are out, and the uterus is starting to contract back to its normal size. The timeline above gives a rough sense of the three stages.

The first stage of labor is the dilation part: your cervix goes from closed to 10 centimeters open. This stage is by far the longest; it can in principle last for days, and it is itself divided into three parts: early labor, active labor, and transition. Early labor is the period where you go from a closed cervix to about 3 centimeters. This stage of labor tends to be comparatively easy, with mild and fairly infrequent contractions. Many women go through at least some of this stage of labor over a period of days or even weeks, often without knowing it.

After this, you move into active labor, which is more intense and typically not possible to ignore. During this period, the cervix dilates from 3 to 7 centimeters. Active labor can be slow or fast, depending on the woman, and usually involves more frequent contractions. The final part of the first stage is called *transition*, and is the period in which the cervix completes the dilation from 7 to 10 centimeters. For most women, this is the most difficult period of labor. Contractions may come every 2 minutes and last 90 seconds, leaving little room to rest between them. On the plus side, transition tends to be short.

It's worth noting that the lines between these stages are a bit blurry, and some OBs prefer simply to separate labor into "early" and "active" labor (i.e., without making a sharp distinction between active labor and transition). What does seem to be generally true is that labor gets more painful as it progresses.

Once you are fully dilated, it's time for the second stage: pushing. This tends to be shorter, although there is a lot of variation. It can be as short as a few minutes (more common for second- or third-time moms) or as long as a few hours. This stage ends when the baby arrives. You might think that this means you are done, but after the baby you still have to deliver the placenta. This typically occurs immediately after the baby, and with all the excitement and hormones it can be a bit of a blur. It can also be surprisingly painful—the doctor will sometimes push on your stomach to get the placenta out—but it's over quickly.

This is a textbook description of labor—it's what you'll see in virtually every pregnancy book, and it's what your doctor will tell you. For me, there were two crucial pieces of information missing. First, I wanted to understand a bit more about these times. They seemed pretty vague—"a few hours," "could be as much as a day," and so on. I understood that there was a lot of variation across women, but that didn't mean I couldn't learn more details.

I also wanted to understand the most common complications during labor. Obviously I knew that things might arise that I wasn't prepared for, but I didn't want to be blindsided by something that I could have seen coming.

Let's start with the timing question.

The first part of labor (the 0 to 3ish centimeters) can take a very long time. There is really no predicting it. Many women dilate to this level over a period of *weeks*, often without noticing. There's no sense worrying about timing here.

Once you hit active labor—and you'll know because the contractions will get more regular, and more painful—the timing is a bit more predictable (although only a bit). The standard story—the one discussed in the leading obstetrics textbook, for example—is that labor should progress at the rate of at least 1 centimeter an hour. Their view is that most women will go faster than this, and, in fact, you should start to worry if you progress more slowly. With this kind of timing we would expect active labor to take 6 hours or less. When I first read this I found it surprising, as nearly everyone I knew had labor that lasted longer than that.

When I looked into it a bit more, this information started to seem a little outdated. The source of this figure is a study of 500 women published in 1955.[1] There is no particular reason to think that women labor more slowly now than they did in the 1950s, but the management of labor has changed, as has our ability to analyze data. Perhaps it is worth revisiting these numbers?

In fact, in a 2002 paper, researchers in Hawaii did just that, studying the labors of 1,300 women and updating the earlier conclusions.[2] Their findings were pretty different. These researchers found that during active labor, women dilate *on average* about 1 to 2 centimeters per hour (note that this is the *average*—the earlier study said that 1 centimeter was the cutoff for being too slow).

This speeds up as you go forward: the average woman will take almost 6 hours to go from 3 to 7 centimeters, but will go from 7 to 10 centimeters in 90 minutes or less (this is that transition period). The newer data also shows that before 7 centimeters, it would not be uncommon for women to go 2 or even 3 hours without *any* apparent change in dilation. This may be helpful to know because going for long periods with no progress can be frustrating and cause women (and sometimes their doctors) to question whether the process will ever progress.

The data on timing actually also answered part of my second question about labor problems. One of the major problems in labor is that the cervix opens too slowly or not at all. This can lead to a need for various interventions (Pitocin, for example) and can be an indication for a C-section if the baby is in distress (for example, if its heart rate is dropping).

The second common labor problem is that women have trouble pushing the baby out in the second stage of labor. This can happen if the baby is very large or Mom's pelvis is very small. It can also happen if Mom is having trouble with knowing how to push—as it turns out, it can be hard to figure out what it means to "push" the baby out. Depending on how far down the baby gets, doctors will sometimes respond to this by performing a C-section, and sometimes by using medical instruments (forceps or a vacuum extractor) to pull the baby out.

A third possibility is that the baby might be facing the wrong way. It's easier (not easy, just easier) to give birth if the baby is facing toward your back. If the baby is facing up (sometimes called *sunny side*), it can be harder to push her out. Which direction the baby is facing can (and often does) change *during* labor, so this is not something you can predict based on prebirth ultrasounds (although you can see what is going on in an ultrasound during labor). Often it won't be clear that this is a concern until you are actually trying to do it. Again, this can increase the chance of a C-section.

This is perhaps a good place for a word on C-sections. C-sections are generally safe, and they are common (about 30 percent of births in the United States). But OBs generally agree, for good reason, that they are not the preferred mode of delivery. A C-section is major abdominal surgery. Recovery varies across women, but is generally slower than after a vaginal delivery.

At some point I was comparing notes with a friend who had an emergency C-section when her labor "stalled out." We were talking about the first moments home with our babies. She said the first thing she did was open up the computer and order another changing table, as she wasn't going to be able to walk up and down the stairs. The first thing Jesse and I did was take a walk to the coffee shop. I actually drove us all home from the hospital. Ultimately, my friend recovered fine, too, but things just moved along more slowly for her.

Having the option to have a C-section if things go wrong is great; this has undoubtedly saved countless lives. But it shouldn't be the first choice for mode of delivery.

One exception to this, probably, is if your baby is *breech*. The majority of babies come out head first; this is the way that birth is designed. In order for this to happen, of course, they have to be head down at the start of labor. Saying a baby is breech means he is in some other position. In fact there is a variety of kinds of breech. Some babies have their butts down and their legs folded up (in diving this would be called a *pike* position; for a fetus, it is referred to as *frank breech*). Others are cross-legged.

Still others have just one leg hanging down. In this case (called *footling breech*), if your water breaks you can sometimes actually feel a foot come out into your vagina. They told us about this in our birthing class and it, more than anything else, really freaked Jesse out. (I probably don't have to say it, but if this happens to you, call 911 right away.)

Before 36 weeks, your baby being breech is absolutely nothing to worry about. Babies move around all the time. Even closer to your due date, it is usually not anything to worry about. Almost all babies will figure out the right positioning on their own and will rotate. At 28 weeks, perhaps 25 percent of babies are breech; by delivery, it's only 3 to 4 percent.[3] Much of this rotation occurs before 32 weeks. In one study in Sweden only about 7 percent of babies were still breech by 32 weeks; half of those turned on their own by delivery.[4] If your baby still hasn't turned around on its own by 37 weeks, there is an option to try to turn the baby manually.

This is called an ECV: *external cephalic version*. The concept is simple. They give you some medicine to relax your uterus, and then try to muscle the baby around by pushing from the outside. Obviously this is all done with extensive monitoring to make sure the baby is handling it well, and at a hospital so that if something does go wrong they can deliver right away. This procedure is successful about half the time, and has limited complications, although it can be very uncomfortable (you might be offered an epidural).[5]

If this doesn't work and your baby is still breech when you get to labor, you will almost certainly have a scheduled C-section. This wasn't always the case, and it is, in fact, *possible* to have a breech baby vaginally (this is especially true for frank breech). But large randomized studies have shown that vaginal delivery of breech babies is slightly riskier than a planned C-section. If you are dead set on a vaginal delivery with a breech baby you'll likely have to search for a provider who is willing to do it.

The other common cause of a scheduled C-section is if you've had one before. Women who have given birth once by C-section are very often advised to have future babies the same way. Having a vaginal birth after a C-section is possible (it's often called a VBAC, for vaginal birth after Cesarean) but not usually the default. I had more than one friend ask: is this recommendation right?

It's actually a bit hard to know. There are no randomized studies.[6] The best we can do is to compare women who had a C-section and planned a vaginal birth to women who had a C-section and planned a repeat C-section. This isn't perfect—the kind of women who want a VBAC may be different from those who are happy to have another C-section—but done right it can be pretty convincing. And studies like this suggest that there are some increased risks to a VBAC.

In one case, researchers studying women in Australia found that women who planned a VBAC had more serious infant complications and a greater likelihood of maternal hemorrhage. Both of these outcomes happened for about 2.5 percent of the women in the VBAC group versus only about 0.8 percent of the planned C-section group.[7] The women in the two groups looked very similar in many ways—age, race, etc.—so we can have some confidence that the choice of delivery mode was responsible for the differences. And this is pretty consistent with other, similar studies.[8]

Without randomized evidence it's hard to be rock solid on this, and, unlike in the breech case, many doctors will be fine with this type of delivery. Because of the possibility of increased risks, though, you do probably want a doctor who has experience with this situation so that she'll know what to do if things start to go awry. If you do decide to attempt a vaginal birth, be prepared: about half of attempted VBACs end in a C-section.

The Bottom Line

- Labor times vary a lot. Average dilation time is 1 to 2 centimeters an hour after active labor starts.

- There are three major categories of labor problems: (1) dilation is too slow, or stops altogether; (2) baby gets stuck, and (3) baby is facing the wrong way, making it harder to push.

- Emergency C-sections are a good option to have, but a C-section should not be your first choice . . .

- . . . unless your baby is breech or (probably) if you've had a C-section before.

To Epidural or
Not to Epidural?

Pain relief during labor has a long history. There is a good reason for this: childbirth is really painful.

Queen Victoria was among the first women to use anesthesia—in her case, inhaled chloroform—during the birth of her seventh child in 1853. She was a huge fan. The use of this type of pain relief spread, although mostly among upper-class women. In the last century, a form of pain relief called *twilight sleep* became more common. Basically, women were given a combination of morphine and another drug (scopolamine), which caused them to be more or less asleep during birth. It's not clear that twilight sleep actually relieved pain, but it did cause women not to remember the birth. The idea is that you go to sleep and wake up with a baby.

Local pain relief—of which the epidural is one version—was first used in the early 1900s; it initially contained cocaine. Modern versions of the epidural (no cocaine) began to gain in popularity in the 1960s, and today the vast majority of labor pain relief is of this type. Narcotic pain relief (like Nubain or Demerol) is occasionally used but much less commonly. This is for two reasons. First, it doesn't work as well—it dulls the pain but doesn't get rid of it—and second, if it is administered late in labor, it can impact the baby's breathing after birth. Narcotics, therefore, tend to be reserved for early labor pain relief.

You probably have some basic sense of how the epidural works. To greatly simplify, it numbs your lower half, which includes the uterus area. Once you're numb, you may not feel contractions at all—the pain during the pushing part of labor is also lessened or eliminated.

An epidural is administered during the first stage of labor—the part where the cervix is dilating. It is sometimes (but not always) turned off during the pushing, because pushing is often harder if you are completely numb. The epidural procedure is pretty straightforward: a needle is inserted into your back, into the membrane that surrounds the spine, and a catheter is threaded in. Anesthesia is delivered through the catheter. This numbs the lower half of your body, either partially or fully, depending on the dose. The procedure itself might sound painful (or just creepy), but they typically give you a local anesthetic first, and most women don't have any pain after that.

The epidural is extremely popular: it was used in about two-thirds of births in the United States in 2008. At the hospital where I had Penelope, the epidural rate is 90 percent. Before I got pregnant, I expected I would use an epidural. Frankly, I thought natural childbirth was for hippies who didn't believe in medicine (to be fair, that *is* one group who favors drug-free childbirth).

In contrast, I love medicine. I'm the first in line to get my kid vaccinated, and I'm constantly berating my mother about her claim that she doesn't "believe" in the flu shot (what would this even mean? I have never gotten a straight answer). So I figured that I'd do the research and sign up for the drugs.

Some of what I learned was quite positive for the epidural.

There do not seem to be serious negative impacts on the baby, which was a relief. But, on the other hand, the evidence convinced me that there is no free lunch for Mom. I came to conclude that the use of an epidural complicates the process of birth, and probably makes the recovery a bit harder (on average). The risks were small, but they were there.

To be clear, there are very good reasons to get the epidural. Well, there is one particularly good reason. It is really, really good pain relief. This is probably not a place where we really need randomized trials, but if you have any doubt, they exist and confirm this claim. In randomized trials, relative to women who received nonepidural pain relief, women who got an epidural reported less pain during labor.[1] If it works as it should, many women have virtually no pain during the dilation part of labor. During the pushing part there is generally some discomfort associated with pressure more than pain, but clearly less than if you were unmedicated.

Because it limits or eliminates the pain, the epidural can also help you get some much needed rest. The pushing part of labor is physically taxing with or without pain relief. Having an epidural can let you sleep for a few hours of labor, and then be at least slightly better prepared for the most physical part.

Figuring out the risks (if any) required more research. Natural childbirth Web sites warned of everything from paralysis to lethargic babies with no ability to nurse. The childbirth class we took at the hospital mentioned nothing about risks, emphasizing only the awesome benefits. It turned out the truth was somewhere in the middle.

This evidence wasn't as hard to come by as I had expected. There are many randomized controlled trials that evaluated the impact of epidurals. The basic design of these studies is very simple. Women entering the study (either before or during labor) were randomly assigned to have an epidural or not. As the assignment was random, the two groups of women were similar in all ways other than the epidural, so researchers could draw conclusions about the impact of the epidural by comparing them.

You might wonder how they get any women to participate in these studies, with the risk of *not* getting into the epidural group looming. The first answer is that in nearly all these studies, both groups got some kind of pain relief. The studies typically compared the epidural to a narcotic like Demerol (not as good as the epidural for pain, but not nothing). As many of the proposed complications of an epidural are not possible complications of narcotics, we can use these data to make comparisons between the epidural and no pain relief.

The second answer is that women were not *required* to stay in their assigned group. A lot did not—as many as half of the women in some studies who were assigned to the nonepidural group ended up getting an epidural anyway.

For research purposes, the authors of studies like these compared the women who were assigned to get the epidural to those who were assigned not to *regardless of their eventual behavior*. This is called an *intent-to-treat* design. In the group assigned an epidural, virtually everyone got one. In the group *not* assigned to the epidural, fewer people got them. Because the epidural was more common in one group than the other, researchers could draw conclusions about its effect even if some people "cheated" on their assigned group!

The studies focused on two things: impacts on the baby and impacts on the mom. It makes sense to start with the baby, as that is almost certainly your top priority. [2]

Primary conclusion: from the standpoint of the baby, the epidural mostly doesn't matter. Babies who are born to moms who have an epidural are no more likely to spend time in the NICU, and no more likely to have low APGAR scores (meaning they are

Epidural and Baby

Positive Impacts: None identified (although that's not the point!)

Negative Impacts: Increased chance of unnecessary antibiotics

No Differences: APGAR score, fetal distress, baby poop before birth, baby time in NICU

not more likely to be "lethargic," which is one concern that is bandied about).

One issue that is often discussed but doesn't have much evidence either way is breast-feeding success. The most recent meta-analysis of epidural impacts identified only one randomized controlled trial on breast-feeding; although that was small, the epidural had no impact on the timing of lactation. At the very least, we can say there is no affirmative evidence that nursing is impacted by the epidural.

The one negative consequence of an epidural for the baby is related to a maternal complication. For some reason (possibly due to the inability to sweat enough when nerves are blocked), women who get an epidural are much more likely to run a fever during labor. The fever is a known side effect of the epidural, but doctors can't tell if it's a *real* fever (due to an infection) or just a side effect. This leads them to react as if Mom has an infection, which often means treating the baby with antibiotics.

In one study, 90 percent of babies born to women with a fever during labor were given antibiotics, versus only 7 percent of babies born to women without a fever. In the end, *none* of the babies in either group actually needed the drugs.[3]

Unnecessary antibiotics are not ideal, but this is a fairly minor complication. The bigger risks of the epidural are for Mom. The epidural changes the labor experience pretty dramatically.

Epidural and Mom

Positive Impacts: Better pain relief

Negative Impacts: Greater use of instruments (forceps or vacuum in delivery), greater use of C-section for fetal distress, longer pushing time (15 minutes), higher chance of baby facing up at birth,* greater use of Pitocin in labor, greater chance of low maternal blood pressure, less able to walk after labor, greater chance of needing a catheter, increased chance of fever during labor

No Differences: Overall C-section rate, length of dilation period of labor, vomiting during labor, long-term backache

* Only marginally significant

The plus of the epidural is pain relief.

There are a number of negatives. The first among these is an increase in the use of forceps or a vacuum extractor during delivery. These are both used to help get the baby out in cases where they seem to be stuck. Forceps are an older technology—basically, they look like giant salad tongs, and they lock around the baby's head to help pull him out. A vacuum extractor works similarly, but with a suction cup applied to the baby's head.

These are both quite safe for the baby, which is kind of amazing when you see them. During the birth of my nephew, my sister-in-law reported that all it took was just *seeing* the vacuum extractor for her to finally push him out (after four hours). But instruments do increase the chance of vaginal tearing for Mom. They can also lead to some bruising around the baby's head, which can look scary but heals quickly.

The epidural seems to lengthen labor just a bit, mainly by lengthening the pushing stage. It also seems to increase the chance that the baby is born face up (the "wrong" way). This might be due to the fact that in most cases once you have the epidural you don't move around much. Without an epidural, you want to move around during labor—your body is telling you to walk, to switch positions, etc. One theory is that this movement is what helps the baby get into the right position for birth. The lack of movement with the epidural makes this harder.

The other big concern for many women is that an epidural will increase the chance of a C-section. The results in the trials for this are ambiguous. On the one hand, on average the studies here show no impact on the C-section rate (10.7 percent for those with the epidural versus 9.7 percent for those without). On the other hand, when we focus on C-sections done for fetal distress (or perceived fetal distress), 3.5 percent of women with an epidural have these, versus 2.4 percent without. This would suggest that *emergency* C-sections are more likely with epidurals.

On net, these results on C-sections seem mixed and more work likely needs to be done to understand this link better. One issue is that the C-section rates in most of these studies are low; in the United States, the current rate is close to 30 percent. It's possible that the impact of the epidural would be different (could be bigger or smaller) in a setting like this where the overall rate is so high.

The epidural also has a bunch of other effects, ones that you might not have even thought about. There is an increase in the use of Pitocin to get labor going. This is true almost by definition because when you get an epidural it slows down contractions.

Pitocin is needed to speed them up again. It also increases the chance of low blood pressure (for Mom) and the need for a catheter. This last one might seem like a big deal, but it's not really: usually the catheter goes in after the epidural and comes out before the epidural is turned off, so you might not even notice.

A final risk is the inability to walk until the epidural wears off. This seems minor—I mean, where are you going?—but I did hear of someone who got out of bed to pick up the baby, didn't realize she was numb, and broke her toe. In truth, this is probably not a common complication.

Of course, there are many things that the epidural doesn't affect, including some you might have been worried about. The first stage of labor (up to the pushing part) is a similar length for those with and without an epidural. Use of an epidural doesn't seem to increase the risk of a long-term backache, which is a possible concern because it's injected near the spine.

There is one final issue that is not included in the preceding lists and that is the postdural puncture headache. Done correctly, the epidural needle goes into the membrane around your spine, not into the spinal fluid itself. Of course, these are right next to each other, and it's possible to accidentally go into the spinal fluid. If this happens, it's called a *wet tap*, and you have about a 40 percent chance of developing a postdural puncture headache in the few days after labor. Basically, it's a really, really terrible headache lasting for several days.

This wet tap is reasonably common: about 1 in 200 procedures, even at a good hospital.[4] It's much more common if you have a doctor who hasn't done many procedures before, so you definitely want to check that you are not getting some resident who's trying his first epidural.

At some point after reading all this, I started to think that the epidural wasn't for me. Jesse was initially skeptical. "It's up to you," he told me, before pointing out that if it were him he'd hook up to the drugs around 36 weeks just so he didn't run the risk of *any* labor pain.

I didn't really need him on board (I mean, if he opposed the plan that would be a problem, but I didn't need him to be excited). But I thought it would help. If there was any doctor pressure, I knew I wouldn't be in a position to advocate for myself, and I wanted him there to do it. So I collected the studies and e-mailed a report.

He wrote back:

> It seems crystal clear that epidural lengthens labor, increases fever risk and worsens fetal position, very likely that it increases instrumentation and probably that it increases C-section.
>
> It's harder for me to judge the headache issue without more hospital-specific information, but I agree it doesn't help the case.

Shortly after this e-mail we went to our one-day birthing class at the hospital. During lunch, over sandwiches and shortbread cookies at Au Bon Pain, we talked about this decision. We agreed that if there were any real risks to the baby, that would make the decision easy, but in truth, there just didn't seem to be any concrete demonstration of that. Despite the various Internet warnings about how this would impede my ability to nurse or to bond with Penelope, the evidence just wasn't there.

This meant the choice was really about me. I'd summarize it as: harder labor versus easier recovery. Jesse put his hands up—this really wasn't his decision. He could see, from an evidence-driven standpoint, why I might choose not to do it. But if it were him, he'd still do it for sure.

In the end, I decided against it—or, at least, I'd try to go without it. This isn't an especially common decision, and some people definitely thought I was crazy. My mother, who had three children in a period when epidurals were not widely used, was especially incredulous. "They have drugs now!" she kept telling me, before launching into a description of her 96-hour unmedicated labor with me, which concluded with (in her telling) four orderlies pushing down on her stomach to get me out.

If given the choice, Mom definitely would have gone with the epidural. For me, it worked out not to. Although the truth is that if I had had my mother's labor experience, I bet I would have gotten it. I was lucky enough that things went pretty smoothly, and quickly (more on that later). This isn't to say it was easy—two hours of pushing was no joke—but I didn't have a lot of second thoughts.

And as difficult as it was, I was right about the recovery. I was up and walking 45 minutes later and I felt great(ish). In economics we say talk is cheap—you can only really figure out what people like by their actions. So what you should really ask is whether I did it again for the second kid. The answer is yes.

There are some pregnancy decisions where I'd look at the evidence and think, *Boy, someone would be crazy to do this differently.* This was not one of those times. It's easy for me to see the case for the epidural. Most women I know had one, and more or less all of them thought that was the right decision. Jane had her son just a few months after Penelope was born. She had read all of my evidence by then, and we'd talked through this a number of times. She was pretty clear at the outset: she saw the risks, she thought about them, but they seemed small and outweighed by the benefits.

In the end, our labor experiences were very similar, minus the pain: 12 hours of labor, no instruments or a C-section, easy recovery, and healthy babies. In fact, I pushed for 2 hours and she for only 30 minutes, exactly the *opposite* of the effect of the epidural in randomized trials. We talked on the phone the day after her son was born and she told me I was crazy not to have the drugs, and that she was happy to contribute a proepidural testimonial to this book.

Same evidence, two different decisions, two happy moms. Knowing what the evidence says doesn't make the decision for you. It just lets you make the decision in an informed way. The only mistake would be to decide one way or the other without thinking. When women report regretting this decision, it is almost always because they felt they were bullied into what their doctor wanted, rather than what they wanted. You're the one pushing the baby out. It's your choice to make.

Natural Pain Relief

If you decide to go (or try) the nonepidural route, there are various forms of natural pain relief. Most of these involve breathing or some kind of visualization—Lamaze, the Bradley Method, Hypnobabies. For the most part, evidence on these is thin for the simple reason that the kind of women who invest in learning these techniques are *particularly* committed to natural childbirth. It certainly will not hurt you to learn breathing, and it may well be effective; we just can't say based on data.

One natural form of pain relief that does have some randomized evidence is aromatherapy. It appears to have no impact on anything.[5] This is not a surprise to me. I can assure you that if you are laboring without drugs, you are not going to care what type of scented candles are in the room.

On the flip side, there *is* a bit of evidence that acupuncture can have an influence here. A few studies have found that acupuncture during labor improves pain management and reduces the use of other drugs.[6] But caution is warranted: the studies are small, and the evidence is somewhat mixed.[7] It's probably not relevant in any case; most hospitals do not have an acupuncturist on staff.

The Bottom Line

- Epidural is very effective pain relief.

- But it increases the chance of some complications for the mother.

Beyond Pain Relief

The decision not to have the epidural led me to wonder about everything else. The epidural is increasingly standard practice during labor—if I didn't want that, were there other standard things I didn't want?

One thing I quickly realized was that, by and large, women who want to avoid the epidural also want to avoid any other medical intervention. The natural childbirth community is negative on basically any medical interventions during labor—the epidural, yes, but also any other drugs during or after labor, fetal monitoring, any movement restrictions, and so on.

The world really seems to contain two groups: those who would like to avoid any medical interventions, and those who embrace whatever is the standard birth practice. I had a strong instinct to want to align completely with one group or the other— I think this must reflect some basic human desire for group identity—but I didn't want to do this blindly. I wanted to do it with evidence.

Ultimately, I came to think there was some intermediate path.

There were times when I definitely agreed with the natural child-birth group—for example, on the topic of episiotomy—but others when I didn't—for example, Pitocin after birth.

I really only got into this because I was planning not to have the epidural, but in the end I came away thinking it was a shame that people seemed to bifurcate so completely. For the most part, the other choices I made about birth were pretty unrelated to pain medication. A routine episiotomy is a bad idea, and that's true with an epidural or not.

In the service of this, I also came to think a birth plan was a good idea. Ours was a bullet-pointed list (with references, naturally). Of course, the name "birth plan" is silly. Once you have been through labor, the idea that you might have planned for it is laughable. Before Penelope was born I talked with a friend who already had two kids who said the plan should be labor for one hour, no pain, baby slides right out. I mean, as long as you're making a plan, why not go for optimism?

OBs and labor-and-delivery nurses also tend to be a little resistant to birth plans, for some of the same reasons. They worry that if you aren't flexible, they won't have the freedom to make decisions that might be necessary in the moment. Also, having seen childbirth before, many doctors are appropriately skeptical of birth plans with details like, "I want 'Somewhere Over the Rainbow' to be playing when the baby is crowning."

But having thought about some of these decisions before labor actually starts is almost certainly a good idea. Writing them down gives you (or at least gave me) something concrete to discuss with the doctor. If you do this far enough in advance, you can ideally have that conversation in a quiet moment at 36 weeks pregnant, rather than between contractions.

The Birth Plan

I really wanted to avoid an induction. In the end, I was probably more worried about this than was necessary. My major concern was that the stronger contractions that come with Pitocin would make it harder or impossible to go without the epidural. I prepared as well as I could to avoid induction for reasons like low fluid or an unresponsive non-stress test. I was prepared to push my doctor to 42 weeks if Penelope was doing well.

The other major reason for an induction (other than real risk to the mother or baby, for which I would of course have acquiesced immediately) is if your water breaks before labor. Television would have you believe that most women start labor with their water breaking. This is wrong. In fact, less than 10 percent of women have their water break before labor. For most women it doesn't happen until quite late in the process.

If your water does break first, you'll often go into labor right away or within an hour or two. With her first child, my friend Heather described an experience where her water broke, and then 30 seconds later she was in such intense pain that she couldn't speak. This is atypical (her daughter was born just 4 hours later—lightning-fast in first-baby terms), but the vast majority of women are in labor within 12 hours of their water breaking.

But if you're not one of these women, standard practice is to induce labor. Most doctors will strongly encourage this. Their big concern is with infection. The water (the fluid in the amniotic sac) protects the baby from exposure to the outside world. Once that protection is gone, you and the baby are subject to infection.

Given my fear of induction, when I went looking for evidence on this I secretly hoped that I'd find that this wasn't a good policy—that infection was no more likely for women who waited to go into labor on their own. In fact, that wasn't what I found: the evidence does seem to support the standard policy.

The one large randomized trial compared a policy of inducing within 12 hours of water breaking to a policy of letting women wait up to 4 days. The study found no difference in C-section rates and no difference in outcomes for babies. However, there was a large difference in maternal infection rates.[1] These rates tend to be increased when doctors do vaginal exams (more opportunity for bacteria to get in), so they are usually best to avoid in this situation.

I concluded that from the standpoint of Penelope's health, it probably didn't matter much. For my own health, though, inducing soon after my water broke was probably a good idea. *Soon* in this case means within 12 hours or so. There is no need to frantically hail a taxi, but if this happened to us, the plan was for us to make our way to the hospital in the not-too-distant future. In the end, this didn't come up.

Oster Birth Plan, Bullet Point 1:

- If water breaks before contractions start, our preference is to wait 12 hours and induce if labor has not started. Unless necessary, digital vaginal exams should be avoided during this period.

After induction, my second big fear was not being able to drink water during labor. I was under the impression that ice chips were the only available sustenance in the delivery room—no water, never mind snacks. I probably also learned this from television. It terrified me. Even during normal times, I drink a somewhat disturbing amount of water. Now I was going to engage in the most physically demanding task of my life, and I was going to do it with just some chips of ice?!

Television is again somewhat apocryphal: some (although not all) doctors will let you have water. But in many cases this is all you are supposed to have. My doctor told me, "You better eat something before you come in, because once you are here we won't let you have anything." I can't put my finger on it, but there seems to be something odd about that statement.

So, what is the logic? The basic fear is *gastric aspiration*, and it's related to why you shouldn't eat, in general, before any operation. If you are under general anesthesia and you vomit, it is possible to inhale your stomach contents into the lungs and suffocate. Pregnant women may be at more risk than the general population for this. In general, this definitely is dangerous, but you might be wondering why this is an issue in labor. Even if you have a C-section, aren't you usually awake? So wouldn't you know if you were vomiting? Is this still an issue?

To figure out the origin of this restriction, we actually have to go back to a time (the first half of the twentieth century) when C-sections were typically performed under a general anesthetic. The source of the ban on food during labor is a 1946 paper in the *American Journal of Obstetrics and Gynecology.* The authors reported that of 44,016 pregnancies at the Lying-In Hospital in New York from 1932 to 1945, there were 66 incidents of gastric aspiration and 2 deaths from suffocation. The authors suggested withholding food during labor.[2]

Fast-forward 64 years: a lot has changed about labor and medical practice in general. C-sections are now performed with local anesthesia 90 percent of the time, so you are typically not asleep. Moreover, even if you are under general anesthesia, our understanding of how that works has improved a lot. The estimated risk of maternal death from aspiration is 2 in 10 million births, or 0.0002 percent.[3] Yes, maternal mortality is terrifying.

But to put this in perspective: this cause accounts for only 0.2 percent of maternal deaths in the United States, mostly among very high-risk women. The perhaps scary truth is that you're more likely to die in a car accident on the way to the hospital than from this cause.

In a review article from 2009, researchers looked at almost 12,000 women who ate and drank what they wanted during labor. Even though some of these women did need emergency C-sections (one of the few times when you might be under a general anesthesia), there were no problems reported associated with aspiration. This is true even for the 22 percent of women who ate solid food.[4]

And yet the ban on food remains. This is despite the fact that having some calories during labor seems to help women keep up their energy.[5]

To summarize: it's unlikely that you'll be under general anesthesia during labor, even if you have a C-section. And if that did happen, the risk of aspiration is vanishingly small. I certainly felt fine with the idea of eating during labor.

I went into labor midday on my due date. I had a small lunch, some yogurt and fruit, before I realized that all that regular cramping meant something. Jesse came home in the middle of the afternoon and decided we needed something more substantial. I got myself an egg and cheese bagel, which I highly recommend as a prelabor meal. My mother recalls having a ham sandwich, which she also reports is a good option.

It was good that I ate at home, because even my relatively lenient OB practice wasn't into the idea of solid foods in the delivery room. This is common: birthing centers might be different, but most hospitals will not allow you to bring much in the way of snacks.

A good alternative, one that we used, is sports drinks and clear juices (I'll never look at yellow Gatorade the same way again). Research shows these to have a similar upside in terms of energy, and none of the (claimed) risks.[6] And many more doctors and hospitals are comfortable with this idea; the risk of complications from aspiration are all due to solid foods. It's still worth talking this through with your doctor. If he subscribes to the ice-chips-only rule, there may be little you can do (short of switching hospitals or sneaking drinks in!).

Planning for juice or sports drinks may be a good idea for another reason: once labor gets going, you probably are not going to feel like eating. Marathon runners don't typically stop for a ham sandwich, and you probably won't want to take a break for one either. When I was about 7 centimeters dilated, Jesse decided he needed a snack. Fortunately for him, to get to the minimum on the bagel delivery, we had bought some extra bagel sandwiches. He took one out: cream cheese, lox, and red onions. It took all my strength to order him out of the room immediately. I was decidedly *not* sorry that the doctor wouldn't let me share.

Oster Birth Plan, Bullet Point 2:

- I will be drinking water and clear fluids during labor.

When Jesse left me to have his snack, he wasn't totally abandoning me. We had brought along a secret weapon: our doula, Melina. I was the one who pushed the doula idea in the first place. Jesse was, again, initially skeptical, but I was the final decision maker in the case of labor. After it was over, we both agreed that having Melina with us was by far the best decision we (I!) made.

My doctor was great, it was mostly nice to have Jesse there (minus the smelly bagel), but at the end of the day I'm convinced that Melina's presence was the reason everything went so smoothly.

I'm not sure I can articulate quite why this was. I can, of course, say what she actually did—she arrived at our house as labor was getting more intense, stayed with us at home, and then came to the hospital with us and stayed until Penelope arrived. She did some back massage during early contractions, and encouraged me to switch positions when I was getting too comfortable (she actually used that phrase once—"You are getting too comfortable on this birthing ball; you need to lie on your side so the contractions are more intense"). But I'm guessing the bigger benefit was just having someone who knew what was going on and who was calm and relaxed.

In fact, this wasn't just my experience. Several randomized controlled trials have suggested that doulas have a large impact on birth outcomes. In one study, couples were randomly assigned to have a doula or not, starting at hospital admission.[7] Women with a doula were half as likely to have a C-section (13 percent versus 25 percent) and less likely to use an epidural (64 percent versus 76 percent).

An older study, published in 1991, showed similar impacts. Women in this study were randomly assigned to have either a supportive doula or an observer in the room who did not help. Women with a doula were less than half as likely to have an epidural, had shorter labor, were about half as likely to have a C-section, and were half as likely to have forceps used in delivery.[8] Remember that these women were randomly assigned, so this isn't subject to the obvious concern that the kind of people who want a doula are the kind of people who especially want natural childbirth.

One interesting thing to note here: many people think a doula is helpful only for people who are trying to go without the epidural. These studies suggest that this is not the case. The C-section rates were lower even among women who used an epidural.

When my daughter finally emerged (after 2 hours of pushing!), Melina was the one who cut the cord (Jesse was afraid he'd mess it up). She stuck around for a while, helped me try to figure out breast-feeding, and finally ran off to another birth. She came by the house a few days later to check on us, another nice feature of many doula arrangements, and was able to confirm that Penelope was actually swallowing when she nursed (I don't know why it was so hard for me to figure this out). One of my biggest fears is that if we have another child, Melina will have moved away or decided she doesn't want a job that requires her to stay up all night. I'm not sure I could do it without her.

Oster Birth Plan, Bullet Point 3:

- Our doula, Melina, will be with us during labor.

If your plan is to avoid the epidural, they tell you to stay home as long as possible. Home tends to be more comfortable, and once you're in the hospital and they start offering you the drugs, people tend to take them. We stuck around in the house until midnight, at which point I'd been in "real" labor for 4 or 5 hours and the contractions were 3 minutes apart and lasting 1 minute. The natural childbirth books tell you that the time to go to the hospital is when you can't smile in the picture you take on your way out the door. Sounds about right.

Our hospital is about 20 minutes away, and Jesse claims I was backseat driving the whole way. (What can I say? Sometimes he needs advice!) When we got there, as at most hospitals, the first thing they did was hook me up to a fetal monitor. This is the same machine used for the non-stress test described earlier.

Usually there are two belts that go around your belly and provide continuous data on the fetal heart rate.

At many hospitals, this isn't optional: you will be hooked up to some form of this monitor the entire time you are in labor (this is true regardless of whether you have an epidural). Sometimes you'll have the option for a portable monitor so you can walk around. If the doctor can't get a good read on the external monitor, they often use an internal monitor. This is threaded up through the cervix and screwed into the baby's scalp. Yes, you read that correctly.

The point of the monitor is to let the doctor see if the baby is in distress. It records the heart rate and lets doctors see how much it dips down during contractions. If it drops too much, they'll give you oxygen, perhaps try to get things moving faster, or (in the extreme) do a C-section. This type of fetal monitoring has become close to universal in the United States: in 2002, 85 percent of women had this during labor.

I have a lot of personal animosity about this monitoring. When we first arrived at the hospital, they left me immobile on this thing for about 40 minutes in triage. Laboring on your back has got to be among the least comfortable positions—my contractions slowed down, and I got cranky. Jesse was furious—he was about to, in his words, "Go Brooklyn" on them when they finally came in to move me upstairs.

Once I was in the actual delivery room they gave me a portable monitor, which in principle allowed me to move around, but this wasn't much better. When I moved around (presumably the point of the monitor being portable!), the straps moved around also. This meant that about every other contraction, the monitor stopped recording the baby. This caused two problems. First, I freaked out. Second, it meant that as I was trying to work through the contraction, the nurse was fiddling around with the straps. Melina finally told them they'd better turn the volume down or she was taking it off.

But let's not have my personal feelings get in the way. Evidence-based decision making is not assisted by personal animosity. And the principle sounds good: shouldn't it be beneficial for the doctor to know what is going on with the baby at all times? They should be able to identify babies who are in trouble further in advance, leading to better outcomes for both Mom and baby. That's the theory, anyway.

The reality is a bit different. In a 2006 review article, researchers compared continuous monitoring, where you are hooked up to the machine all the time, to intermittent or occasional listening. Intermittent listening is typically done with a stethoscope or a fetal Doppler (like the one they use in your doctor's office at your normal prenatal visits). Every little while (20 minutes, an hour, etc.) the doctor or nurse checks the baby's heartbeat. The advantage of the continuous monitoring, in principle, is that it might identify babies who are in trouble more quickly, because it's measuring the heart rate all the time.

The review article found that women who underwent continuous monitoring were much more likely to have interventions. They were 1.6 times as likely to have a C-section. If you focus in particular on C-sections that were done because of a concern about the heart rate, you find that women with continuous monitoring were 2.4 times as likely to have a C-section for this particular reason. Use of instruments (forceps or a vacuum) was also more likely for women with continuous monitoring.[9]

In principle, this outcome could be good or bad. If the continuous monitoring is doing a better job of identifying babies at risk, then that's a good thing. If so, we'd expect the baby health outcomes to be better with continuous monitoring. This is not the case. There was no difference across babies in APGAR scores, admissions to the NICU, length of time spent in the NICU, or fetal death. The one place that researchers found a difference was in neonatal seizures—these were more likely in the group without continuous monitoring—but they occurred in only 7 of 32,000 births, so the overall risk level is very low.

Based on this evidence, both this review and the most commonly used OB textbook suggest that continuous monitoring isn't necessary or even a very good idea for most women. It seems like what is happening is that doctors overreact to patterns they see in the heart rate when the baby is not actually in distress. It's almost as if there is *too much* information. You might imagine that every baby, no matter how well the birth is going, has a few moments when her heart rate dips. If you aren't watching all the time, you don't see this, and that's fine. If you are watching, you conclude something is wrong, and it's off to the OR.

Despite the evidence, and the fact that the American Congress of Obstetricians and Gynecologists doesn't recommend this for low-risk pregnancies, this type of monitoring is increasingly non-negotiable at many hospitals. I certainly wasn't able to talk my way out of it even though my hospital was fairly progressive. It's worth asking whether your OB is okay with intermittent monitoring, where you are hooked up to the machine for 10 or 20 minutes every hour but free to move around the rest of the time. This is a bit more invasive than listening to the baby with a Doppler, but it may give you more freedom and let you avoid some of the negative outcomes of continuous monitoring.

Oster Birth Plan, Bullet Point 4:

• Intermittent (ideal) or mobile fetal monitoring

My labor was pretty close to textbook. I was 5 centimeters dilated when I arrived at the hospital, 4 hours later I was fully dilated, and 2 hours after that Penelope was here. If you're doing the division, you'll see that is a bit faster than 1 centimeter an hour. That's right around what the old "standard" labor curve would view as the slow end of normal. As I said before, that is pretty outdated, and many labors go more slowly, or at least more fitfully, than that. That is *fine, normal*.

But if your labor is going really slowly, and really has stalled, there are two common interventions. One is to use Pitocin, the same drug you would use to induce labor in the first place. This speeds up the frequency and intensity of contractions, which moves labor along. The second is to break your water if it hasn't already broken—sometimes called an amniotomy. This is done with a device that looks very much like a crochet hook. Like the Pitocin, this tends to speed things up.

Evidence suggests that either or both of these interventions (sometimes they are done together) will speed up labor, and they do not generally have other complications (no changes in C-section rates, or bad outcomes for the baby).[10] Doctors will often do the amniotomy first, as your water is going to break sometime anyway, and move to drugs if that isn't successful.

I actually did have a version of this. Near the end of labor, I was about 9.5 centimeters dilated and the OB pointed out that my water wasn't fully broken. She said if they went ahead and broke it the rest of the way, I would be fully dilated and ready to go. This was fine with us—it was in the birth plan—and I was glad we had thought about it in advance, as I wasn't in my most rational decision-making place at that point.

Something I didn't realize before labor is that your doctor is actually not there most of the time. For hours it was just Jesse, me, Melina, and Nurse Tera. I've been told that if I had had the epidural, the nurse wouldn't even have been there most of the time. The doctor swoops in when you are ready to push. She will basically take over at that point.

Usually everything goes fine, but this is the part of labor

Oster Birth Plan, Bullet Point 5:

- If labor progression is slow *during active labor,* our preference for augmentation is (in this order): (1) amniotomy
(breaking water) and (2) Pitocin.

when the physical doctor skills can really come in handy. The
big concern here is that the baby will get stuck. Until you try
it, it's hard to know how things are going to work out. It's difficult
to visualize the size of Mom's pelvis (contrary to what I thought,
having observably good "birthing hips" doesn't really relate), and
ultrasound estimates of the baby's size are often misleading.

Most babies don't actually get stuck, but it is *very* common for
women, especially with their first baby, to have some vaginal
tearing. At some point, doctors got the (I guess not crazy) idea
that babies would be less likely to be stuck, and there would be
less tearing, if they just widened the opening a little bit. This led
to adoption of a procedure called an episiotomy.

The idea is simple: the doctor cuts an incision in the perineum
(the area between your vagina and anus) to make it easier for the
baby to come out. This was also supposed to make it easier to fix:
a clean cut can be stitched more easily than a tear. This procedure
used to be extremely common: it was used in about 60 percent of
births in the United States in 1979.

But even as this procedure was in wide usage, people wondered: was this really such a great idea? Think about trying to
tear a piece of fabric in half. You'll find that you have a much
easier time doing that if you start by cutting it a bit. But by the
same logic, maybe you could actually make things *worse* by cutting the vagina before the baby came out. As it turns out, these

concerns are well placed: most of the time an episiotomy does more harm than good.

The sanity of this intervention has been tested in a number of randomized trials.[11] The trials typically compare two policies: one in which doctors perform episiotomies as a routine matter for almost everyone, versus a policy in which they do so only if they feel it is absolutely necessary. In a review of these trials, this difference in policies makes a big difference: 72 percent of women in the "routine" group had an episiotomy, versus only 27 percent in the "only if absolutely necessary" group.

Outcomes in these trials were worse for the routine episiotomy group. This group was more likely to have an injury to their perineum, more likely to need stitches, and (in one small study) had more blood loss. They also had more pain at the time of leaving the hospital and more complications with healing. One argument often made in favor of routine episiotomy is that it prevents really bad tearing. However, these studies showed *no* differences in the frequency of severe trauma in the two groups.

The one outcome that favored the routine episiotomy group was injury toward the front of the vagina, which makes sense because the episiotomy makes it more likely that any tearing will happen toward the back. However, the outcomes on healing, infection, and blood loss suggest that the increased risk of this type of trauma is strongly outweighed by the decrease in risk of other injury.

Fortunately, likely as a result of this strong evidence against routine use of this procedure, episiotomies have dropped from around 60 percent in 1979 to only about 25 percent by 2004.[12] We put this in the birth plan just as a precaution, but we also made sure to discuss it with the OB before labor. If she had said anything about doing this in a routine way, I would have run in the other direction. There is no reason for this to be done routinely, and if your OB feels differently, I might look for one who has read the medical literature in the last twenty years!

Oster Birth Plan, Bullet Point 6:

- No routine episiotomy

Up to this point, for the most part I found myself nodding right along with natural childbirth people. I had a lot of skepticism about the fetal monitoring, the snack restrictions, the episiotomy. But one place where I really broke with the whole no-drug camp was in the question of Pitocin after birth.

Significant blood loss after birth is one of the most common complications of delivery; in the developing world, it is a common cause or contributor to maternal mortality. In the developed world, better medical technologies make the mortality risks vastly lower, but significant blood loss still requires treatment. It has long been known that drugs that cause uterine contractions (like Pitocin) can be used to *stop* blood loss once it starts, but more recently, randomized trials have noted that using these drugs *before* any blood loss occurs can dramatically decrease the risk of this complication.[13]

This is perhaps not surprising, as Pitocin is the synthetic form of oxytocin, the hormone that is released when you start breastfeeding. Presumably, evolution designed the system this way for a reason: you have the baby, and when you start nursing you get a surge of hormones to help your uterus contract and prevent bleeding. The natural system is great, but the synthetic form of the hormone also helps.

There are some risks associated with this intervention. The same randomized trials that show decreases in hemorrhage also show increases in blood pressure (for Mom), more pain after birth, and more vomiting. These are good to know about, although I would guess they probably won't change your ultimate thinking on this, and they certainly didn't change mine.[14]

If you have had an IV, you probably won't even notice this being administered: the doctor will just stick it in the IV and that'll be the end of it. When I had Penelope, however, my IV came out during the pushing, so they had to give me a shot to the leg. This resulted in the worst leg cramp I've ever had. It's a testament to how quickly you forget the pain of labor that I remember this as the worst part of the whole thing. Jesse assures me it was definitely *not* the worst.

Oster Birth Plan, Bullet Point 7:

- Pitocin in the third stage is fine if necessary/recommended.

A final word. Mostly, childbirth doesn't go quite like you expect it to. I was told that labor would start with contractions 5 to 10 minutes apart and gradually get closer. Instead, they started 2 minutes apart and stayed that way for 12 hours. I expected to push for 20 to 30 minutes—an hour at the absolute most!—but found myself still pushing 2 hours in. One friend went to her OB at 39 weeks only to be told that her fluid was low and her baby was breech and she needed an immediate C-section. Another spent 5 hours moving from 5 to 6 centimeters, finally got an epidural, and was fully dilated and pushing 45 minutes later.

There are just too many possibilities to have any real plan. The best you can do is have some idea of what's coming, and think through the most likely scenarios. Be prepared, but don't be committed. In the end, maybe something will happen you aren't expecting, and you'll have to go with that. You can't prepare for everything.

At the end of the day, it really doesn't matter where she comes out of, what drugs you did or didn't have, what procedures were or were not done. Birth plan, shmirth plan. What matters is that she is a person, and she's yours.

The Bottom Line

- *Broken water:* Induce if labor doesn't start on its own within 12 hours.

- *Eating and drinking during labor:* Probably should be allowed, although most hospitals still will not let you have solid foods, and you probably aren't going to want them anyway. Do bring some Gatorade to keep your energy up.

- *Doula:* Having a doula decreases the chance of a C-section and of using an epidural. Recommended.

- *Continuous fetal monitoring:* There's no evidence it's effective. If intermittent monitoring is available, do that.

- *Labor augmentation:* Labor can progress slowly, and does for many women. The 1-centimeter-per-hour rule is probably a bit optimistic. But there are limited downsides to augmentation; both breaking the water and use of Pitocin tend to speed up labor without increasing C-section rates or other complications.

- *Episiotomy:* **Not a good idea.**

- *Pitocin after birth:* Useful in preventing postpartum hemorrhage. Recommended.

The Aftermath

The moments of Penelope's arrival were a blur. There was a flurry of activity. Penelope had her hand up by her face during the birth (apparently this is why it took so long to push). The doctor pulled her halfway out and whipped her arm around (Jesse describes it as: "She took the arm off, turned the baby around, and put it back on"). She was out. They dropped her on top of me, suctioned her mouth, and she started to yell. They cut the cord. They wrapped her in something and I held her.

The whole process is a bit abrupt and overwhelming: all of a sudden there is another person there. When Penelope arrived, Jesse and I both cried. But this isn't the only possible reaction. One father I know was so overwhelmed holding his son for the first time, he started listing all the state capitals.

Once you hold the baby a bit (or your partner does, if you have had a C-section), they'll take her to the other side of the room—for weight, measurement, footprints, and so on. Of course this is all only the beginning of the decisions you'll have to make. Circumcision, breast-feeding—whether to do it and for how long—sleep training, vaccinations, day care versus nanny, and on

and on. Jesse keeps pointing out that eventually we'll have to figure out who will teach Penelope to drive (it will be me; he is a
terrible driver). For the most part, these are left for another day.
But there are a few things that happen *in* the delivery room—
decisions you'll have to make before you have the baby.

Delayed Cord Clamping

I will admit that I hadn't even heard of this until our doula mentioned that we might want to think about it. When I did a little
more research, it seemed to come up in natural childbirth circles.
Then, when Penelope was about seven months old, the *Economist* published an article about it. I guess that's how you know
the idea has entered the mainstream.

The idea is that rather than cutting the cord right away, you
should wait, usually just a couple of minutes, so that the baby can
"reabsorb" some of the blood from the placenta. The natural
childbirth view is that it's artificial to cut the cord right away: tra-
ditionally the baby would have been placed on the mother first.

When I looked into it a bit more, I found that whether this is
a good idea depends on the baby's prematurity, and the conditions into which he is born. For premature infants (those born
before 37 weeks of pregnancy), delayed cord clamping seems to
be a good idea.[1] It roughly halves the need for a blood transfusion
for anemia, and has an even bigger effect on the need for blood
transfusions for low blood pressure. Basically, it seems like preterm babies need more blood, and this is an easy, natural way to
get it to them.

For babies born full term, the evidence is more mixed, but
increasingly it also seems to favor delayed clamping.[2] On the plus
side, just as with preterm infants, delayed clamping is associated
with higher iron levels (less anemia) that persist for at least 6

months. On the negative side, some studies (although not all) have shown that delayed clamping is associated with a 40 percent increase in the risk of somewhat serious jaundice. This all makes sense: jaundice happens when the baby is a little slow to get rid of bilirubin, a byproduct of red blood cells. When the baby gets more blood from the cord, this problem gets worse while the anemia problem improves. In the preterm infant, the need for blood is greater, so you get the positives without the negative.

This is where the location of birth matters. Anemia is not very common in the United States because our nutrition is fairly good. This means that delayed clamping is perhaps less beneficial. In the developing world, anemia is much more common, and the benefits likely outweigh the risks. The ultimate question for you is whether you are worried more about anemia or more about jaundice. We are lucky that in the United States both conditions are extremely treatable, so you're unlikely to make a big mistake either way.

Vitamin K Shots

It is standard to give babies vitamin K supplementation within the first hours after birth. The purpose is to prevent bleeding disorders. A deficiency of vitamin K can cause unexpected bleeding in up to 1.5 percent of babies in the first week of life (the bleeding could come from the umbilical area, be prompted by a needle stick, or be internal). It can also cause bleeding later, between 2 and 12 weeks of age. Although it's rare (perhaps 1 in 10,000 babies), this second manifestation is much worse: it often causes severe neurological damage or death.

Supplementation with vitamin K is very good at preventing this. It's typically given through a shot, although it can also be given orally. Evidence suggests that both are effective, but the oral dosing slightly less so.[3] Vitamin K supplementation has been standard since the 1960s. Unless you ask about it, you probably will not even know the doctor is doing it; it'll just be one of the several things they do when they are cleaning up the baby.

Despite the fact that it's standard, this shot is not free of controversy. In the early 1990s, several studies from the United Kingdom suggested that these shots might be linked to an increased risk of childhood cancer. In one study, researchers compared 33 children who developed cancer before age ten to 99 children who did not. They looked at many factors and found that vitamin K shots were one thing that was more common among the children with cancer.[4]

The same researchers followed up with a slightly larger study (195 children with cancer) and again found that vitamin K shots were more common among the children with cancer than those who were not sick.[5] The authors argued that, in particular, vitamin K *shots* were associated with cancer, while vitamin K given orally seemed to make no difference.

Although this may give you pause, further work has not provided support for this claim. For one thing, other researchers pointed out that because childhood cancer is, mercifully, rare, if there was any connection between vitamin K and cancer, we would expect to see huge increases in childhood cancers after these shots became standard in the 1960s, and we do not.[6] Further, attempts to replicate the study by other researchers have not shown similar results.[7]

The American Academy of Pediatrics responded to this controversy in 2003 with a review of the debate and reaffirmed their position that vitamin K shots should be standard. They argued that the benefits in preventing bleeding were large, and the best available work suggested no link with cancer.[8] This seems correct to me. Although the specter of childhood cancer is scary, the evidence is simply not there to support a link to vitamin K supplementation, and we know for sure that bleeding disorders are a risk.

Antibiotics in the Eye

Historically, untreated sexually transmitted infections were a major source of infant blindness. When babies were exposed to gonorrhea or chlamydia in the vagina during birth, their eyes sometimes became infected, leading to partial or complete loss of sight. It turns out that treatment with (historically) silver nitrate and (now) antibiotics can prevent a large portion (perhaps 80 to 90 percent) of these infections.[9] The treatment is given as drops or cream in the eye; there are generally no complications other than a bit of redness and irritation. It's likely you won't even notice.

This treatment is obviously a good idea if you have (or might have) an untreated sexually transmitted infection. That is increasingly less common, in part because it's routine to test for these during pregnancy, which makes it a bit less clear what the benefit is. Many countries in Europe have dropped this standard practice with no increase in blindness. Having said that, there are no apparent problems with this treatment and you probably won't be given a choice. Most states in the United States mandate it. Although in principle you might be able to opt out, it's not easy.

Cord-Blood Storage

Cord-blood storage is not mandatory by any means. Nor is it free. But starting around the middle of pregnancy you'll be bombarded with offers from private cord-blood banks. In our experience, they don't like to take no for an answer; after we decided against this we continued to receive updated offers, with increasingly low prices, right up until Penelope's birth. I'm surprised they were not at the hospital when we checked in, offering a last-ditch deal.

If you do decide to store your cord blood, the blood from the umbilical cord will be drained into a container for storage, and taken away and frozen for later use. It typically costs a few thousand dollars.

Why would you do this? The idea is that stem cells from cord blood might be useful in treating some diseases. If you have one of several rare blood disorders (you would know if you do), there can be significant value to this option. For people without these particular conditions, the most likely current benefits lie in being an alternative to a bone marrow transplant for leukemia. It is important to note: your child cannot typically use his *own* cord blood if he gets sick. The value is in it being used by a sibling. If one of your children is sick, a sibling's cord blood could possibly be used.

So there is some potential benefit to cord-blood storage, at least to your family overall, but in numerical terms it's tiny. One study suggested that only about 3,000 transplants of cord blood to children had been done worldwide overall. Most of these—the vast majority—were done with cord blood from someone unrelated. The data suggest that for families without a blood disorder, the chance of using the cord blood they banked is about 1 in 20,000.[10]

The big sales pitch that these companies make is that although the uses *right now* are fairly limited, there are going to be many more uses for stem cells in the future. That may well be correct. However, you want to keep in mind that advances are being made in other technologies also. For example, scientists are making progress on developing stem cells from regular cells.[11] Once this is possible, it is likely to be a lot better than getting stem cells from cord blood. They are not there yet, but there is no particular reason to think that the technology for making stem cells will advance more slowly than the technology for using them.

A final note: this whole discussion is about *private* cord-blood banking. Another related option is to donate your baby's cord blood to a public blood bank. The chance that your child's cord blood could be used by someone else outside your family is much greater than the chance that it would be used within your family. This is especially true if you are a member of an ethnic or racial minority. Public cord-blood donation is also free, or close to it. If you're interested, this is something that is typically coordinated through the hospital where you deliver your baby.

The Bottom Line

- *Delayed cord clamping:* a good idea if the baby is born before 37 weeks. If the baby is full term, it's up to you to trade off the (possibly) higher risk of jaundice with the lower risk of anemia.

- *Vitamin K shots:* effective at preventing bleeding, and the claims that they increase the risk of cancer are unsubstantiated.

- *Eye antibiotics:* probably not necessary if you don't have an untreated sexually transmitted infection, but legally mandated in most states and without any obvious downside.

- *Cord-blood banking:* very unlikely to be useful for your family given current technology. Future technology is difficult to predict. Public cord-blood banking is worth considering.

Home Birth: Progressive or Regressive? And Who Cleans the Tub?

One of the most common discussion topics on the pregnancy chat board I visited was the Ricki Lake documentary *The Business of Being Born*. The movie is best described as a propaganda piece about home birth, with the surprise addition of full frontal Ricki Lake nudity at the end. Ricki and the various other interviewees in the movie rail against what they see as the overly medicalized process of birth. After all, they argue, women have been giving birth for thousands of years at home, so why do we need to involve hospitals?

I have a very hard time with this argument. When I'm not researching pregnancy, much of my work focuses on the developing world. At one point, I spent several weeks in Nepal, working on a project about menstruation and schooling. While there, I toured a maternity hospital. To say that it was bare bones would be a generous exaggeration. Women gave birth inside the hospital, but within the first hour they were moved into a giant room, all together, open to the outside. Their families staked out small areas in the room and were *cooking*. That's right. You have your baby, and then go lie on a pallet on the floor in an outdoor room, surrounded by other people, everyone cooking lentils and rice. Then a bunch of researchers from the United States traipses through on a tour.

You would think this is a prime example of a situation in which one would rather have the baby at home. Yet hospitals like that one are the reason that the maternal mortality rate in Nepal is a third of what it was thirty years ago, and the infant mortality rate is less than half. This is true for many reasons: the ability to have an emergency C-section if necessary, antibiotics to fight infection, Pitocin to ward off maternal hemorrhage, doctors who know how to maneuver a baby out of the birth canal if her shoulders get stuck, and so on. In the developing world, giving birth in a hospital is much, much safer than doing so at home.

To be direct about it: it's true that women have been giving birth at home for millions of years, but a lot of them, and many more of their babies, died.

Having said all this, giving birth at home in a birthing tub in New York City is a far cry from a bed in rural Nepal. Backup medical intervention is close, and modern technology can be brought to you. This means it might not be appropriate to look at changes over time in the developing world and draw conclusions about the United States. After all, home births are much more common in Europe than in the United States, and Europe has significantly lower infant mortality rates.

And the truth is, I can sort of see the appeal. When I was in labor, the process of traveling to the hospital and waiting in triage was among the most unpleasant parts. I objected to the fetal monitoring, and to the fact that they made me get an IV put in just in case (then never used it). It might have been nice to simply stay at home and lounge around in the bathtub. My friend Dwyer had a home birth. She had an amazing experience with no complications and has turned into a bit of a home-birth fanatic.

So, might a home birth be for you? The easy answer, just based on the numbers, is probably not: fewer than 1 percent of women in the United States have a home birth.[1] An only slightly more nuanced answer is not if you want pain medication. There is no epidural option at your house.

In addition, this isn't going to be an option if you are high risk (for example, if your baby is breech, if you are having twins, if you have gestational diabetes, etc.). Unless you live in an especially home-birth-friendly area (Berkeley, perhaps), it will be difficult or impossible to find a midwife who will attend a birth of this type. It's just too risky.

This leaves low-risk women with healthy pregnancies who have no interest in an epidural. If you happen to be in this group, and are even considering a birth at home, you'll want to think carefully about weighing the pros of a home birth against the cons.

The Pros

For women who are committed to avoiding an epidural, an often-voiced fear is that the hospital will "force" them to get one or that in the midst of a particularly difficult period of labor they'll give in and ask for medication. Although the hospital cannot actually force you to have an epidural, they may suggest it more often than you'd like. A home birth gets around this issue: it's a way to commit to your decision without having to constantly reinforce it to other people.

A second thing in the "pro" category is that most women are probably more comfortable and more relaxed at home, which could make labor faster and easier. Even the nicest delivery rooms in hospitals are not that nice; your home is almost certainly more relaxing and Zen-like. In addition, if you have the baby at home, you avoid a hospital stay later. This could be good or bad, but may be a plus for some women.

Finally, there is hard evidence that, on average, births at home are associated with fewer interventions and an easier recovery. Comparing low-risk births that were planned to take place at home (regardless of where they actually took place) versus those that were planned to take place at the hospital, researchers found that the planned home births had less monitoring, fewer epidurals, fewer episiotomies, less use of forceps, and a lower C-section rate. They also had fewer vaginal tears and lower infection rates.[2]

The Cons

Jesse and I never seriously considered a home birth, but when we talked about this issue in an academic sense, the main downside he could not see past was the mess. Where does the water from the tub go? he kept wondering. Would he have to clean it himself? Wouldn't that be messy? He finally made me ask Dwyer. It turns out, in case you are also wondering: the midwife deals with it and most of the water gets flushed.

So one "con" of home births is the mess, but that's a surmountable issue. The much bigger concern is what happens if something goes wrong. In a life-or-death situation for you or the baby, surgery or other serious intervention is an ambulance ride away, not in the room next door.

The main thing you need to know, therefore, is what the chance is that something will go wrong. There are two ways things can go wrong. Something could go a little wrong, and you could end up going to the hospital and having the baby there. Or something could go a lot wrong, and either you or the baby could be seriously injured or die. This second scenario could happen at home, or it could happen if you decide to go to the hospital but are too late.

A Little Wrong: Hospital Transfer

A large percentage of planned home births do not happen at home. Estimates vary, but one summary suggests that as many as *a third* of mothers planning first-time home births end up at the hospital. For women who have already had a child, it is only about 10 percent, perhaps because only women who have had a fairly smooth birth the first time would plan this for their second child (or because the second tends to be a bit easier).[3]

This means that if you are a first-time mom and you do plan a home birth, there is a 30 percent chance that you'll end up having to transfer to the hospital anyway. This could happen for any number of reasons: because you change your mind, because the midwife decides labor is going too slowly, or because the baby is in distress.

If you do end up transferring to the hospital during labor, chances are this is going to be *more* disruptive than if you had planned to go in the first place, as you may not be prepared (or packed!). This means that when you think about a home birth, you want to think about whether you'd rather have a 70 percent chance of having the baby at home and a 30 percent chance of transferring to the hospital frantically at the last minute or a 100 percent chance of going to the hospital in a (somewhat) relaxed manner. You also want to think about how far away the hospital is. The farther you are from a hospital, the more likely that something going a little wrong could turn into something going a lot wrong.

A Lot Wrong: Injury or Death

The last-minute hospital transfer that results in a healthy baby and mom is disruptive but not disastrous. But lurking in the background is a much bigger risk: that you won't know to go to the hospital in time, or that things will happen so quickly that you can't get there. And if this happens you fear the worst: that you or the baby could be injured or die. This is not some abstract fear. Births happen every day, but they can be dangerous.

We know that hospital births save lives in very poor countries. However, the medical literature has struggled to answer the question of whether the same is true in rich countries like the United States. From a research standpoint, there are two barriers to getting a good answer here. First, women who plan to have their babies at home aren't really like women who plan to give birth in a hospital. Home-birth women tend to be rich, highly educated, and white. Babies born to women in this group are less likely to die regardless of where they are born, so it's misleading to compare them to a random sample of babies born in the hospital.

Even more problematic, the women who actually *end up* giving birth at home are those who have such an easy birth that they don't end up as part of the 30 percent who go to the hospital. So of course if you compare women who have their babies at home to other women, they will almost always look like their babies do better, but that's *very* misleading.

This second issue is a pretty big deal. To get around it, the best studies of this compare women based on their *planned* birth location, rather than on their *actual* birth location. In these studies the home-birth group includes women who thought they'd have a home birth but ended up in the hospital. By comparing women based on their plans, the researchers at least avoid the most basic problem that only the "easy birth" people end up having their babies at home. They are still left with the other problem, that the kind of woman who wants to have her baby at home may be different in other ways.

Studies of this issue are mostly small, but a recent review article combined a large number of them to attempt to draw some conclusions about the risks (or lack thereof) of home birth.[4] This study got a lot of attention when it came out: it was published in a good medical journal, appeared to be comprehensive, and was critical of home birth. Based on the results in the study, the American Congress of Obstetricians and Gynecologists (the main source for pregnancy recommendations) suggested that women be told that the risk of infant death is 2 to 3 times higher with home birth than in a hospital. Although the risk of infant death in either group is really, really tiny (2 in 1,000 versus 0.9 in 1,000), this increase may be big enough to convince a lot of women that home birth is not for them.

The home-birth lobby went *ballistic* when this article came out. They attacked it from all sides: the authors were biased, they didn't understand statistics, they included too many studies—no, too few! Medical journals sometimes publish comments on their papers, but these are typically limited to one or two per paper. The journal published at least six comments on this, plus an author reply. They also convened an independent panel to rereview the evidence in the paper, an extremely unusual step.

It seems likely that regardless of its merits, this paper would have generated a lot of attention, and probably a lot of criticism. But in this case, as it turns out, at least some of the criticism seemed well founded. One problem with the paper is that it simply had a lot of small mistakes—which is probably more common in research papers than you realize; most research doesn't get this kind of scrutiny, so little mistakes never come out. The authors made some calculation errors, errors in their statistical analysis, and so on. These problems may lead you to question the competence of the authors, but correcting the errors didn't ultimately change the paper's conclusions.

A much bigger issue with this paper lies in the fact that it combined studies that measured infant mortality in different ways. One way to measure infant deaths is with "perinatal mortality." This includes stillbirths and deaths within 28 days of life. A second way to measure infant death is "neonatal mortality," which includes *only* deaths up to 28 days of life among babies born alive.

If home births increase deaths after birth, they should increase both the neonatal and perinatal mortality rate. If they increase deaths during the birth process, they should increase the perinatal mortality but not the neonatal mortality.

What the authors actually found is a bit odd. When they analyzed perinatal mortality they found that home births did not impact deaths. But when they looked at neonatal mortality they found that home births did increase deaths, by a lot. Think about what this would mean. We can explain these results only if home births *decreased* stillbirths. But why would that be?

In fact, when I looked a bit more at the paper I quickly realized what was going on. The paper is a meta-analysis, meaning it combines a lot of studies. Some of those studies reported results on perinatal mortality and some of them on neonatal mortality. *The two sets of results come from different studies.* Which to believe? It's not clear, although the more reassuring perinatal mortality data has 500,000 births, versus only about 50,000 for the neonatal mortality results.

Do we trust the studies of perinatal mortality more (perhaps because there are 10 times as many people in them)? Or do we take the more cautious route and make our choice as if the neonatal mortality results were correct?

Unfortunately, despite all the attention, this study seems inconclusive. How can we learn anything without knowing more about which of the underlying research we should trust more? In fact, the original papers behind this study are mostly no better. Consider two studies in the Netherlands, one published in 2009 and one in 2010, both of which evaluated the safety of home birth (or midwife-assisted birth).[5] One study found no increased risk of infant death among home births and the other found a 2 to 3 times higher risk of infant death. There is no obvious reason for the difference.

For every study that found an increased risk of death in home births (for example, one in Washington state from the early 1990s), there is one that found no increased risk (for example, a study from British Columbia in the same period).[6] And new studies are coming out all the time. As this book was coming together, another large study in the United Kingdom found that births at home or in midwife units had similar risks to hospital births, although births at home in particular were slightly riskier for women having their first child.[7]

And at the same time, as useful as these studies are, we probably want to combine them with some logic. To be frank, it seems very unlikely that there isn't some added risk to home birth. They may be very rare, but there are situations in which it matters whether you are 10 minutes away from the operating room or 30 seconds away. All the added monitoring and procedures in the hospital, while perhaps annoying, do not *increase* the risk of death. Add these together and we must conclude there is some additional risk; how much is not something we can address with logic alone, and thus far it's really not something answered in the medical literature.

Everything here has focused on risks to the baby. What about risks to you? Although a number of studies report on risks to the mother, there is really no conclusive statistical evidence. Luckily for those of us who live in rich countries, maternal mortality is really, really rare: in the United States, it's about 11 in 100,000 births. This is so unusual that basically no study will be large enough to detect whether there are differences in death rates. This doesn't mean there is no increased risk (although it could mean this), just that the baseline risks are so low that we can't really tell if they are increased.

Home-Birth Attendants

If you think through the pros and cons and still decide a home birth might be for you, the most important follow-up decision you'll need to make is about who will be there with you. Obviously you aren't going to deliver the baby yourself (this is *really* not recommended, although some people do it, usually by accident). Home births are typically not supervised by a physician. Most commonly, people use a midwife.

Most midwives you will encounter have some type of training. But not all midwife training is created equal. At the top of the pyramid are the *certified nurse-midwives* (CNMs). This credential means the midwife is trained in both nursing and midwifery, has at least a bachelor's degree, and is certified by the American College of Nurse-Midwives. There are other categories as well. *Certified professional midwives* have varying types of training (they likely do not have a nursing degree), but have passed a rigorous test from a second midwife association called the North American Registry of Midwives. Finally, *direct entry midwives* typically have some training but not a college degree, and are not licensed by one of the national accreditation groups.

Put simply, if you are going to have a home birth, you want it to be with someone who has as much training as possible, and this generally means a certified nurse-midwife. You can be sure that person has serious medical training—a nursing degree—as well as accreditation from the most rigorous accreditation agency.

The importance of midwife training comes through in the medical literature. Even that recent paper that concluded home birth was risky was careful to note that there was no evidence of increased risk for home births that were supervised by certified nurse-midwives. Why does it matter? The more training the person has, the better she will be at addressing the problem if something does go wrong, and identifying if and when you need to head to a hospital. In addition, the best trained midwives will have experience and ability at infant resuscitation. This means that if something does go wrong with the baby, she can step in until an ambulance arrives.

So, Would You Do It?

Dwyer, my Park Slope home-birth friend, pushed me to think about a home birth when I got pregnant a second time. As she pointed out, I did it once without drugs and without complications, and wouldn't it be nice not to have to spend all that time in the car and waiting around at the hospital? And there was a (small) part of me that did see the appeal. And yet. For me, the possibility of the risk is just too large. I decided I'd rather try to have the kind of birth I wanted in a hospital than admit the tiny chance of a complication. In the end, my son was born in a birthing center room inside the hospital, complete with a tub and a promise of limited fetal monitoring (not that it mattered, since we only made it to the hospital fifteen minutes before the baby arrived). When I talked to Dwyer about it, she said that for her it's just the opposite: she accepted that despite picking the best midwife she could find and doing things as safely as possible there was still some very small increased risk. For her, this was outweighed by the nearly certain benefits of fewer interventions.

The Bottom Line

- If you don't want any pain medication, there are some pros to home birth. There are fewer C-sections, less instrument delivery, easier recovery for Mom, and less tearing.

- If you haven't done this before, there is about a 30 percent chance you'll end up in the hospital anyway.

- Some studies suggest that mortality risks are higher with home birth, others do not. Risks are low in any case.

- If you do decide to go this route, make sure you choose as experienced a midwife as possible, ideally a certified nurse-midwife, who has had nursing, midwifery, and infant resuscitation training.

Epilogue

Because Penelope was born first thing in the morning, our insurance covered two nights in the hospital. On the second night, Jesse went home to sleep. We decided that it was best for us to face the first day at home alone with at least one well-rested parent. They took Penelope to weigh her and do a few tests, and returned with her at two A.M. I was sleeping. The nurse switched on the light and rolled the bassinet in; in addition to Penelope, the bassinet had a little sign: BREAST-FEEDING ONLY.

"We weighed her," the nurse said, "and she's lost eleven percent of her body weight. Our limit is ten percent, so you'll have to start supplementing with formula. If you don't, you probably won't get to take her home tomorrow."

After fourteen hours of labor, barely any sleep, and the ridiculous hormone surge that comes with having a baby, I was in no position to argue. As committed as I was to breast-feeding, the mom part of my brain couldn't fathom the idea of going home without Penelope. And yet the researcher was still there in the back of my mind, telling me that 11 percent and 10 percent seemed pretty much the same—how did they come up with this rule?

I felt like an idiot. I was so focused on pregnancy, I didn't even think to read chapter 20 of my obstetrics textbook: "The Neonate." Never mind doing any actual research. Now I was being outmatched by some arbitrary cutoff rule.

And as I was thinking this, the nurse was setting up something called a "Supplemental Nursing System," in which a bottle of formula hangs from the bed and a tube is taped to your breast so the baby can "think" she is nursing when she is really getting formula. It was awkward and uncomfortable and again I kicked myself for not researching nipple confusion. Was this any better than a bottle? It seemed *more* confusing!

What's the big deal, anyway? How bad was it if Penelope got some formula? Is there any difference between "exclusive" breast-feeding and just "mostly" breast-feeding? Was I costing my child her chance at going to college by allowing her two ounces of formula?

Of course, Penelope survived the introduction of some formula and we made it through the night (you will have to stay tuned to find out if she loses out on Ivy League admission). In the morning, I called Jesse. "Bring the textbook," I told him, "and my computer." The real decision making was just beginning.

• • •

Quick Reference: OTC and Prescription Drugs

Allergies

Both Claritin and Benadryl are Category B drugs. A large-scale study of the association between Benadryl and 324 birth defects found no evidence that use of this drug early in pregnancy increased the risk. Although there were some cases in which particular birth defects were more common among women who took Benadryl, given the number of defects analyzed, these associations almost certainly occurred by chance.[1]

Claritin has similar safety evidence. A study done in Israel of women exposed to the active ingredient in Claritin found no evidence of an increased risk of any birth defects.[2]

This information may also be useful to those women who find Benadryl helpful as a sleep aid. Go right ahead—the same Category B ranking applies to that use as well.

Antibiotics

Not all antibiotics are safe during pregnancy, but there are many good options. General studies of the safety of antibiotics suggest that the majority carry no increased risk for birth defects. Macrobid, for example, is Category B. So is Zithromax. In the latter case several small studies suggest no evidence of birth defects, although the Category B ranking probably relies on general evidence of antibiotic safety.[3] Amoxicillin is another Category B option; so is penicillin. The latter has probably the strongest evidence of safety.[4]

It's worth noting that this is one area where it's probably quite a lot worse to avoid the drugs. If you have an infection, it can pass to the baby and cause serious damage. Hoping that an infection will go away on its own just so you can avoid antibiotics is almost certainly more dangerous than taking the drugs.

Antidepressants

Most SSRIs (Prozac, Zoloft, etc.) are Category C. There is some suggestive but inconsistent evidence of heart defect risk from exposure.[5] Paxil has been more strongly linked to heart defects, so it's a Category D drug. If possible, it should be avoided and your doctor might suggest a switch to another SSRI. For any of these drugs there does seem to be a risk of a withdrawal-like condition in newborns whose mother took these drugs late in pregnancy.

This is a case where you are undoubtedly going to end up weighing the emotional risks of going off the drugs for a time against the possibility of a small risk to the baby. There is no one answer to this and it surely depends on the severity of your illness before starting an antidepressant.

Heartburn and Acid Reflux

These drugs are especially important given that these issues tend to flare up during pregnancy—heartburn in particular. If you have serious acid reflux prior to pregnancy, the most common treatment is Prilosec, a proton pump inhibitor. This drug is Category C. This is one of those cases where Category C might be too cautious. This drug is fairly widely studied and seems to be quite safe. Two cohort studies in Europe and a meta-analysis of 134,000 births in the United States show no evidence of increased risk of birth defects.[6]

For the less serious cases a popular over-the-counter option is Pepcid AC. This is Category B; studies of first trimester exposure in Europe show no evidence of risk.[7] The simplest solution when you are not pregnant also works here: antacids (Tums and the like) are not absorbed into your bloodstream, so they are fine to take. In fact, because they contain calcium, which pregnant women tend to get too little of, some research suggests that women should be encouraged to take antacids even if they are not having heartburn.[8]

High Blood Pressure

There are many types of treatment for high blood pressure, and within each drug category are many different options. It's worth looking up your particular drug. The two most commonly prescribed drugs in this area are Prinivil (an ACE inhibitor) and Norvasc (a calcium channel blocker).

Prinivil is Category D (Category C in the first trimester). A reasonably large, well-controlled study shows evidence of higher rates of birth defects for first trimester exposure. Second and third trimester exposure is linked to renal failure.[9] I think, if anything, the FDA is not cautious enough on this: I would avoid it even in the first trimester.

Norvasc is Category C, and seemingly fairly safe. Several studies, including a fairly large one in Europe, show no increased risk of birth defects.[10] There is some correlation with higher rates of preterm birth, although this is very likely due to the fact that people with high blood pressure, regardless of treatment, are more likely to have premature babies.

High Cholesterol

If you are on any drug to lower your cholesterol your doctor may take you off it during pregnancy for the simple reason that cholesterol is important for fetal development so it's not an especially good idea to keep your levels down during pregnancy.

Largely for this reason, the two most popular cholesterol drugs—Lipitor and Zocor (generic names atorvastatin and simvastatin, respectively)—are Category X. You will almost certainly be taken off these during pregnancy and put back on after. However, unlike in the case of Accutane discussed in chapter 4, accidental exposure to these drugs does not seem to be a significant issue. Although some studies done in animals show evidence of harm, two small studies in humans show no evidence of an increased risk of birth defects.[11]

Painkillers

Over-the-counter options include acetaminophen (Tylenol), ibuprofen (Advil), and aspirin. Most other brand names are simply combinations of these active ingredients (for example: Excedrin migraine is acetaminophen, aspirin, and caffeine). Evidence on acetaminophen is summarized in chapter 4. It's a Category B drug with widely demonstrated evidence of safety.

Ibuprofen (Advil) is Category C. One large-scale study of exposure (not a randomized study, but an observational one) analyzed the relationship between taking ibuprofen in the first trimester and a large number of birth defects. This study found some evidence of a link with spina bifida and cleft lip, but the impacts were small and, given the number of outcomes considered, it seems possible they occurred by chance.[12]

Of these three, aspirin is the one with the most concern: it's a Category D drug. Aspirin in combination with alcohol has been shown to cause birth defects in mice and dogs.[13] At least one small study in humans from the 1970s showed an increased risk of stillbirth.[14] However, a larger study from the same time period showed no increase in birth defects or mortality.[15]

If you need something stronger, you'll most likely be prescribed Vicodin or hydrocodone, both of which are Category C. These are discussed in more detail in chapter 4; although evidence is a little mixed, most of it suggests these are safe.

Notes

Introduction

1. M. Gentzkow and J. Shapiro, "Preschool Television Viewing and Adolescent Test Scores: Historical Evidence from the Coleman Study," *Quarterly Journal of Economics* 123, no. 1 (2008): 279–323.

Chapter 1: Prep Work

1. Federation CECOS, D. Schwartz, and M. J. Mayaux, "Female Fecundity as a Function of Age," *New England Journal of Medicine* 306, no. 7 (1982): 404–6.

2. E. Magann et al., "Pregnancy, Obesity, Gestational Weight Gain, and Parity as Predictors of Peripartum Complications," *Archives of Gynecology & Obstetrics* 284, no. 4 (2011): 827-36.

3. S. Choi, I. Park, and J. Shin, "The Effects of Pre-Pregnancy Body Mass Index and Gestational Weight Gain on Perinatal Outcomes in Korean Women: A Retrospective Cohort Study," *Reproductive Biology & Endocrinology* 9, no. 1 (2011): 1–7.

4. N. J. Sebire et al., "Maternal Obesity and Pregnancy Outcome: A Study of 287,213 Pregnancies in London," *International Journal of Obesity & Related Metabolic Disorders* 25, no. 8 (2001): 1175.

5. C. J. Brewer and A. H. Balen, "The Adverse Effects of Obesity on Conception and Implantation," *Reproduction* 140, no. 3 (2010): 347–64.

6. L. A. Nommsen-Rivers et al., "Delayed Onset of Lactogenesis Among First-Time Mothers Is Related to Maternal Obesity and Factors Associated with Ineffective Breastfeeding," *American Journal of Clinical Nutrition* 92, no. 3 (2010): 574–84.

7. R. Ruager-Martin, M. J. Hyde, and N. Modi, "Maternal Obesity and Infant Outcomes," *Early Human Development* 86 (2010): 715–22.

Chapter 2: Data-Driven Conception

1. A. J. Wilcox, D. D. Baird, and C. R. Weinberg, "Time of Implantation of the Conceptus and Loss of Pregnancy," *New England Journal of Medicine* 340 (1999): 1796–99.
2. A. J. Wilcox, C. R. Weinberg, and D. D. Baird, "Timing of Sexual Intercourse in Relation to Ovulation—Effects on the Probability of Conception, Survival of the Pregnancy, and Sex of the Baby," *New England Journal of Medicine* 333, no. 23 (1995): 1517–21.
3. M. Jurema et al., "Effect of Ejaculatory Abstinence Period on the Pregnancy Rate after Intrauterine Insemination," *Fertility and Sterility* 84, no. 3 (2005): 678–81.
4. C. Gnoth et al., "Cycle Characteristics After Discontinuation of Oral Contraceptives," *Gynecological Endocrinology* 16, no. 4 (2002): 307–17.
5. C. L. Nassaralla et al., "Characteristics of the Menstrual Cycle After Discontinuation of Oral Contraceptives," *Journal of Women's Health* 20, no. 2 (2011): 169–77.
6. I. Wiegratz et al., "Fertility After Discontinuation of Treatment with an Oral Contraceptive Containing 30 Mg of Ethinyl Estradiol and 2 Mg of Dienogest," *Fertility and Sterility* 85, no. 6 (2006): 1812–19.
7. D. Mansour et al., "Fertility After Discontinuation of Contraception: A Comprehensive Review of the Literature," *Contraception* 84 (2011): 465–77.
8. M. Guida et al., "Efficacy of Methods for Determining Ovulation in a Natural Family Planning Program," *Fertility and Sterility* 72, no. 5 (1999): 900–904.
9. R. J. Fehring, "Accuracy of the Peak Day of Cervical Mucus as a Biological Marker of Fertility," *Contraception* 66, no. 4 (2002): 231–35.
10. J. E. Robinson, M. Wakelin, and J. E. Ellis, "Increased Pregnancy Rate with Use of the Clearblue Easy Fertility Monitor," *Fertility and Sterility* 87, no. 2 (2007): 329–34.

Chapter 3: The Two-Week Wait

1. Steven Gabbe, Jennifer Niebyl, and Joe Leigh Simpson, *Obstetrics: Normal and Problem Pregnancies* (Philadelphia, PA: Churchill Livingstone, 2007).
2. A. J. W. Wilcox, "Incidence of Early Loss of Pregnancy," *New England Journal of Medicine* 319, no. 4 (1988): 189.

Chapter 4: The Vices: Caffeine, Alcohol, and Tobacco

1. C. O'Leary et al., "Prenatal Alcohol Exposure and Language Delay in 2-Year-Old Children: The Importance of Dose and Timing on Risk," *Pediatrics* 123, no. 2 (February 2009): 547–54.

2. K. Sayal et al., "Binge Pattern of Alcohol Consumption During Pregnancy and Childhood Mental Health Outcomes: Longitudinal Population-Based Study," *Pediatrics* 123, no. 2 (February 2009): e289–96.

3. E. L. Abel, "Fetal Alcohol Syndrome: The 'American Paradox,'" *Alcohol and Alcoholism* 33, no. 3 (May–June 1998): 195–201.

4. B. L. Anderson et al., "Knowledge, Opinions, and Practice Patterns of Obstetrician-Gynecologists Regarding Their Patients' Use of Alcohol," *J Addict Med* 4, no. 2 (June 2010): 114–21.

5. M. Robinson et al., "Low-Moderate Prenatal Alcohol Exposure and Risk to Child Behavioural Development: A Prospective Cohort Study," *BJOG* 117, no. 9 (August 2010): 1139–50.

6. F. V. O'Callaghan et al., "Prenatal Alcohol Exposure and Attention, Learning and Intellectual Ability at 14 Years: A Prospective Longitudinal Study," *Early Human Development* 83, no. 2 (February 2007): 115–23.

7. R. Alati et al., "Intrauterine Exposure to Alcohol and Tobacco Use and Childhood IQ: Findings from a Parental-Offspring Comparison Within the Avon Longitudinal Study of Parents and Children," *Pediatric Research* 64, no. 6 (December 2008): 659–66.

8. A. Skogerbo et al., "The Effects of Low to Moderate Alcohol Consumption and Binge Drinking in Early Pregnancy on Executive Function in 5-Year-Old Children," *BJOG* 119, no. 10 (September 2012): 1201–10.

9. B. Sood et al., "Prenatal Alcohol Exposure and Child Behavior at Age 6 to 7 Years: Dose Response Effect," *Pediatrics* 108, no. 2 (2008): e34.

10. K. Albertsen et al., "Alcohol Consumption During Pregnancy and the Risk of Preterm Delivery," *American Journal of Epidemiology* 159, no. 2 (January 15, 2004): 155–61; F. Parazzini et al., "Moderate Alcohol Drinking and Risk of Preterm Birth," *European Journal of Clinical Nutrition* 57, no. 10 (October 2003): 1345–49; J. Henderson, R. Gray, and P. Brocklehurst, "Systematic Review of Effects of Low–Moderate Prenatal Alcohol Exposure on Pregnancy Outcome," *BJOG* 114 (2007): 243–52.

11. Henderson, Gray, and Brocklehurst, "Systematic Review of Effects of Low–Moderate Prenatal Alcohol Exposure on Pregnancy Outcome," *BJOG* 114 (2007): 243–52.

12. A. Andersen et al., "Moderate Alcohol Intake During Pregnancy and Risk of Fetal Death," *International Journal of Epidemiology* (2012): 1–9.

13. N. Maconochie et al., "Risk Factors for First Trimester Miscarriage—Results from a UK-Population-Based Case–Control Study," *BJOG* 114 (2007): 170–86.

14. M. Robinson et al., "Low-Moderate Prenatal Alcohol Exposure and Risk to Child Behavioral Development: A Prospective Cohort Study," *BJOG* 117, no. 9 (August 2010): 1139–50.

15. O'Leary et al., "Prenatal Alcohol Exposure and Language Delay in 2-Year-Old Children."

16. B. Larroque and M. Kaminski, "Prenatal Alcohol Exposure and Development at Preschool Age: Main Results of a French Study," *Alcoholism: Clinical and Experimental Research* 22, no. 2 (1998): 295–303.

17. A. Streissguth et al., "IQ at Age 4 in Relation to Maternal Alcohol Use and Smoking During Pregnancy," *Developmental Psychology* 25, no. 1 (1989): 3–11.

18. Albertsen et al., "Alcohol Consumption During Pregnancy and the Risk of Preterm Delivery"; Parazzini et al., "Moderate Alcohol Drinking and Risk of Preterm Birth."

19. A. Nehlig and G. Debry, "Potential Teratogenic and Neurodevelopmental Consequences of Coffee and Caffeine Exposure: A Review of Human and Animal Data," *Neurotoxicology and Teratology* 16, no. 6 (1994): 531–43.

20. A. Pollack et al., "Caffeine Consumption and Miscarriage: A Prospective Study," *Fertility and Sterility* 93, no. 1 (January 2010): 304–6.

21. D. A. Savitz et al., "Caffeine and Miscarriage Risk," *Epidemiology* 19, no. 1 (January 2008): 55–62.

22. Source: http://www.mayoclinic.com/health/caffeine/AN01211.

23. B. H. Bech et al., "Coffee and Fetal Death: A Cohort Study with Prospective Data," *American Journal of Epidemiology* 162 (2005): 983–90.

24. X. Weng, R. Odouli, and D. Li, "Maternal Caffeine Consumption During Pregnancy and the Risk of Miscarriage: A Prospective Cohort Study," *American Journal of Obstetrics and Gynecology* 198: 279.e1–279.e8.

25. J. D. Peck, A. Leviton, and L. D. Cowan, "A Review of the Epidemiologic Evidence Concerning the Reproductive Health Effects of Caffeine Consumption: A 2000–2009 Update," *Food and Chemical Toxicology* 48, no. 10 (2010): 2549–76.

26. Weng, Odouli, and Li did find a link with non–coffee consumption, although it was less significant ("Maternal Caffeine Consumption During Pregnancy and the Risk of Miscarriage"); Bech et al. did not find a link, although they did find one with coffee consumption ("Coffee and Fetal Death: A Cohort Study with Prospective Data").

27. L. Fenster et al., "Caffeinated Beverages, Decaffeinated Coffee and Spontaneous Abortion," *Epidemiology* 8, no. 5 (September 1997): 515–23.

28. B. H. Bech et al., "Effect of Reducing Caffeine Intake on Birth Weight and Length of Gestation: Randomized Controlled Trial," *BMJ* 334, no. 7590 (February 2007): 409.

29. J. L. Mills et al., "Moderate Caffeine Use and the Risk of Spontaneous Abortion and Intrauterine Growth Retardation," *JAMA* 269, no. 5 (February 3, 1993): 593–97.

30. B. H. Bech et al., "Coffee and Fetal Death: A Cohort Study with Prospective Data," *American Journal of Epidemiology* 162 (2005): 983–90.

31. S. Cnattingius et al., "Caffeine Intake and the Risk of First-Trimester Spontaneous Abortion," *New England Journal of Medicine* 343, no. 25 (December 2000): 1839–45.

32. M. H. Aliyu et al., "Association Between Tobacco Use in Pregnancy and Placenta-Associated Syndromes: A Population-Based Study," *Archives of Gynecology and Obstetrics* 283, no. 4 (April 2011): 729–34.

33. V. W. Jaddoe et al., "Active and Passive Maternal Smoking During Pregnancy and the Risks of Low Birthweight and Preterm Birth: The Generation R Study," *Paediatric and Perinatal Epidemiology* 22, no. 2 (March 2008): 162–71.

34. P. Fleming and P. S. Blair, "Sudden Infant Death Syndrome and Parental Smoking," *Early Human Development* 83, no. 11 (November 2007): 721–25.

35. G. Salmasi et al., Knowledge Synthesis Group, "Environmental Tobacco Smoke Exposure and Perinatal Outcomes: A Systematic Review and Meta-Analyses," Acta Obstet Gynecol Scand 89, no. 4 (2010): 423–41.
36. Aliyu et al., "Association Between Tobacco Use in Pregnancy and Placenta-Associated Syndromes."
37. J. Lumley et al., "Interventions for Promoting Smoking Cessation During Pregnancy" (Review), *Cochrane Database of Systematic Reviews* 4, article no. CD001055 (October 18, 2004).
38. Ibid. (*Note: Because this summarizes studies of the impact of quitting partway through pregnancy, we can conclude that this is helpful*); Jaddoe et al., "Active and Passive Maternal Smoking During Pregnancy and the Risks of Low Birthweight and Preterm Birth." (*Note: Because the largest impacts here are at 25 weeks, we can conclude that if you smoked at 18 weeks but not at 25 weeks your baby would be better off*).
39. T. Coleman, C. Chamberlain, and J. Leonardi-Bee, "Efficacy and Safety of Nicotine Replacement Therapy for Smoking Cessation in Pregnancy: Systematic Review and Meta-Analysis," *Addiction* 106, no. 1 (January 2011): 52–61.
40. C. Oncken et al., "Nicotine Gum for Pregnant Smokers: A Randomized Controlled Trial," *Obstetrics & Gynecology* 112, no. 4 (October 2008): 859–67.

Chapter 5: Miscarriage Fears

1. S. Tong et al., "Miscarriage Risk for Asymptomatic Women After a Normal First-Trimester Prenatal Visit," *Obstetrics & Gynecology* 111, no. 3 (2008): 710–14; G. Makrydimas et al., "Fetal Loss Following Ultrasound Diagnosis of a Live Fetus at 6–10 Weeks of Gestation," *Ultrasound in Obstetrics & Gynecology* 22, no. 4 (2003): 368–72; J. L. Mills et al., "Incidence of Spontaneous Abortion Among Normal Women and Insulin-Dependent Diabetic Women Whose Pregnancies Were Identified Within 21 Days of Conception," *New England Journal of Medicine* 319, no. 25 (1988): 1617–23.
2. L. Regan, P. R. Braude, and P. L. Trembath, "Influence of Past Reproductive Performance on Risk of Spontaneous Abortion," *BMJ* 299, no. 6698 (1989): 541–45.
3. G. Makrydimas et al., "Fetal Loss Following Ultrasound Diagnosis of a Live Fetus at 6–10 Weeks of Gestation."
4. Y. Ezra and J. G. Schenker, "Abortion Rate in Assisted Reproduction—True Increase?" *Early Pregnancy: Biology and Medicine* 1, no. 3 (1995): 171–75.
5. L. M. Hill et al., "Fetal Loss Rate After Ultrasonically Documented Cardiac Activity Between 6 and 14 Weeks, Menstrual Age," *Journal of Clinical Ultrasound* 19, no. 4 (1991): 221–23.
6. Steven Gabbe, Jennifer Niebyl, and Joe Leigh Simpson, *Obstetrics: Normal and Problem Pregnancies* (Philadelphia, PA: Churchill Livingstone, 2007); Y. Sorokin et al., "Postmortem Chorionic Villus Sampling: Correlation of Cytogenetic and Ultrasound Findings," *American Journal of Medical Genetics* 39, no. 3 (1991): 314–16.

7. J. L. Mills et al., "Incidence of Spontaneous Abortion Among Normal Women and Insulin-Dependent Diabetic Women Whose Pregnancies Were Identified Within 21 Days of Conception," *New England Journal of Medicine* 319, no. 25 (1988): 1617–23; D. H. Gilmore and M. B. McNay, "Spontaneous Fetal Loss Rate in Early Pregnancy," *Lancet* 1, no. 8420 (1985): 107.

8. P. R. Wyat et al., "Age-Specific Risk of Fetal Loss Observed in a Second Trimester Serum Screening Population," *American Journal of Obstetrics & Gynecology* 192, no. 1 (2005): 240–46.

Chapter 6: Beware of Deli Meats!

1. http://www.cdc.gov/mmwr/preview/mmwrhtml/rr4902a5.htm.

2. A. J. C. Cook et al., "Sources of Toxoplasma Infection in Pregnant Women: European Multicentre Case-Control Study," *BMJ* 321, no. 7254 (2000): 142–47.

3. http://www.cdc.gov/mmwr/preview/mmwrhtml/rr4902a5.htm.

4. V. Janakiraman, "Listeriosis in Pregnancy: Diagnosis, Treatment and Prevention," *Review of Obstetrics and Gynecology* 1, no. 4 (Fall 2008): 179–85.

5. Steven Gabbe, Jennifer Niebyl, and Joe Leigh Simpson, *Obstetrics: Normal and Problem Pregnancies* (Philadelphia, PA: Churchill Livingstone, 2007).

6. A. Bakardjiev, J. Theriot, and D. Portnoy, "Listeria Monocytogenes Traffics from Maternal Organs to the Placenta and Back," *PLOS Pathogens* 2, no. 6 (2006): e66.

7. Joshua Cohen et al., "A Quantitative Analysis of Prenatal Intake of Prenatal Methyl Mercury Exposure and Cognitive Development," *American Journal of Preventative Medicine* 29, no. 4 (2005): 353–65.

8. http://www.fda.gov/food/foodsafety/product-specificinformation/seafood/foodbornepathogenscontaminants/methylmercury/ucm115644.htm.

9. Cohen et al., "A Quantitative Analysis of Prenatal Intake of n-3 Polyunsaturated Fatty Acids and Cognitive Development," *American Journal of Preventative Medicine* 29, no. 4 (2005): 366–74.

10. J. R. Hibbeln et al., "Maternal Seafood Consumption in Pregnancy and Neurodevelopmental Outcomes in Childhood (ALSPAC Study): An Observational Cohort Study," *Lancet* 369, no. 9561 (2007): 578–85.

11. S. A. Lederman et al., "Relation Between Cord Blood Mercury Levels and Early Child Development in a World Trade Center Cohort," *Environmental Health Perspectives* 116, no. 8 (2008): 1085–91.

Chapter 7: Nausea and My Mother-in-law

1. M. A. Klebanoff et al., "Epidemiology of Vomiting in Early Pregnancy," *Obstetrics and Gynecology* 66, no. 5 (1985): 612–16; R. L. Chan et al., "Maternal Influences on Nausea and Vomiting in Early Pregnancy," *Maternal & Child Health Journal* 15, no. 1 (2011): 122–27.

2. Klebanoff, et al., "Epidemiology of Vomiting in Early Pregnancy."

3. R. L. Chan, et al., "Severity and Duration of Nausea and Vomiting Symptoms in Pregnancy and Spontaneous Abortion," *Human Reproduction* 25, no. 11 (2010): 2907–12.

4. R. Lacroix, E. Eason, and R. Melzack, "Nausea and Vomiting During Pregnancy: A Prospective Study of Its Frequency, Intensity, and Patterns of Change," *American Journal of Obstetrics & Gynecology* 182, no. 4 (2000): 931–37.

5. Ibid.

6. N. M. Lee and S. Saha, "Nausea and Vomiting of Pregnancy," *Gastroenterology Clinics of North America* 40, no. 2 (2011): 309–34.

7. L. Dodds et al., "Outcomes of Pregnancies Complicated by Hyperemesis Gravidarum," *Obstetrics & Gynecology* 107, no. 2 (2006): 285–92.

8. Chan et al., "Severity and Duration of Nausea and Vomiting Symptoms in Pregnancy and Spontaneous Abortion."

9. A. Matthews et al., "Interventions for Nausea and Vomiting in Early Pregnancy," *Cochrane Database of Systematic Reviews* 9, article no. CD007575 (2010).

10. Carl Zimmer, *"Answers Begin to Emerge on How Thalidomide Caused Defects,"* New York Times, March 15, 2010.

11. G. Koren et al., "Effectiveness of Delayed-Release Doxylamine and Pyridoxine for Nausea and Vomiting of Pregnancy: A Randomized Placebo Controlled Trial," *American Journal of Obstetrics & Gynecology* 203, no. 6 (2010): 571.e1–7.

12. Ibid.

13. P. M. McKeigue et al., "Bendectin and Birth Defects: I. A Meta-Analysis of the Epidemiologic Studies," *Teratology* 50, no. 1 (1994): 27–37.

14. Z. Bártfai et al., "A Population-Based Case-Control Teratologic Study of Promethazine Use During Pregnancy," *Reproductive Toxicology* 25, no. 2 (2008): 276–85; L. A. Magee, P. Mazzotta, and G. Koren, "Evidence-Based View of Safety and Effectiveness of Pharmacologic Therapy for Nausea and Vomiting of Pregnancy (NVP)," *American Journal of Obstetrics and Gynecology* 186 (2002): S256–61.

15. Magee, Mazzotta, and Koren, "Evidence-Based View of Safety and Effectiveness of Pharmacologic Therapy for Nausea and Vomiting of Pregnancy (NVP)."

Chapter 8: Prenatal Screening and Testing

1. The figures for risk here come from Steven Gabbe, Jennifer Niebyl, and Joe Leigh Simpson, *Obstetrics: Normal and Problem Pregnancies* (Philadelphia, PA: Churchill Livingstone, 2007). This textbook also provided good general background for this chapter.

2. www.bookofodds.com: a good general source for figuring out what probabilities really mean.

3. F. C. Wong and Y. M. Lo, "Prenatal Diagnosis Innovation: Genome Sequencing of Maternal Plasma," *Annual Review of Medicine* (2015).

4. H. Zhang et al., "Non-invasive Prenatal Testing for Trisomies 21, 18 and 13: Clinical Experience from 146,958 Pregnancies," *Ultrasound in Obstetrics & Gynecology* 45, no. 5 (2015): 530–8.

5. G. E. Palomaki et al., "DNA Sequencing of Maternal Plasma to Detect Down Syndrome: An International Clinical Validation Study," *Genetics in Medicine* 13, no. 11 (2011): 913–20.

6. In practice, the risk that will eventually be reported to you by your doctor depends on exactly what software she uses for her calculations and what risk cutoff she uses. The numbers here are based on a 1-in-300 cutoff. Detection rates are very similar for a study in the United States called the FASTER trial, which is slightly older and smaller (30,000 individuals). F. D. Malone et al., "First-Trimester or Second-Trimester Screening, or Both, for Down's Syndrome," *New England Journal of Medicine* 353, no. 19 (2005): 2001–11.

7. K. O. Kagan et al., "Screening for Trisomy 21 by Maternal Age, Fetal Nuchal Translucency Thickness, Free Beta-Human Chorionic Gonadotropin and Pregnancy-Associated Plasma Protein-A," *Ultrasound in Obstetrics & Gynecology* 31 (2008): 618–24.

8. Malone et al., "First-Trimester or Second-Trimester Screening, or Both, for Down's Syndrome." *New England Journal of Medicine* 353, no. 19 (2005): 2001–11.

9. K. Spencer and K. H. Nicolaides, "A First Trimester Trisomy 13/Trisomy 18 Risk Algorithm Combining Fetal Nuchal Translucency Thickness, Maternal Serum Free β-hCG and PAPP-A," *Prenatal Diagnosis* 22, no. 10 (2002): 877.

10. K. Sundberg and J. Bang, "Randomised Study of Risk of Fetal Loss Related to Early Amniocentesis Versus Chorionic Villus Sampli," *Lancet* 350, no. 9079 (1997): 697.

11. NICHD National Registry of Amniocentesis Study Group, "Midtrimester Amniocentesis for Prenatal Diagnosis," *JAMA* 236, no. 13 (1976): 1471–76, 1976. Cited in Steven G. Gabbe, Jennifer R. Niebyl, and Joe Leigh Simpson, *Obstetrics: Normal and Problem Pregnancies : 4th Edition* (New York: Churchill Livingstone, 2002).

12. A. Tabor et al., "Randomized Controlled Trial of Genetic Amniocentesis in 4606 Low-Risk Women," *Lancet* 327, no. 8493 (1986): 1287–93.

13. K. A. Eddleman et al., "Pregnancy Loss Rates after Midtrimester Amniocentesis," *Obstetrics & Gynecology* 108, no. 5 (2006): 1067–72.

14. A. O. Odibo et al., "Revisiting the Fetal Loss Rate After Second-Trimester Genetic Amniocentesis: A Single Center's 16-Year Experience," *Obstetrics & Gynecology* 111, no. 3 (2008): 589–95; V. Mazza et al., "Age-Specific Risk of Fetal Loss Post Second Trimester Amniocentesis: Analysis of 5043 Cases," *Prenatal Diagnosis* 27, no. 2 (2007): 180–83.

15. A. B. Caughey, L. M. Hopkins, and M. E. Norton, "Chorionic Villus Sampling Compared with Amniocentesis and the Difference in the Rate of Pregnancy Loss," *Obstetrics & Gynecology* 108 (2006): 612–16; *Obstetrics & Gynecology* 109, no. 1 (2007): 205–6 (print).

16. Randomized data on this is difficult. There is one Cochrane review that summarizes this. They found similar miscarriage risks for transabdominal CVS versus amniocentesis, but this is based on only a single study. It is also complicated by the fact that CVS occurs earlier in pregnancy. Z. Alfirevic, F. Mujezinovic, and K. Sundberg, "Amniocentesis and Chorionic Villus Sampling for Prenatal Diagnosis," *Cochrane Database of Systematic Reviews* 3 (2003).
17. A. O. Odibo et al., "Evaluating the Rate and Risk Factors for Fetal Loss After Chorionic Villus Sampling," *Obstetrics & Gynecology* 112, no. 4 (2008): 813–19.
18. D. Driscoll, M. Morgan, and J. Schulkin, "Screening for Down Syndrome: Changing Practice of Obstetricians," *American Journal of Obstetrics and Gynecology* 200, no. 459 (2009): e1–e9.

Chapter 9: The Surprising Perils of Gardening

1. A. J. C. Cook et al., "Sources of Toxoplasma Infection in Pregnant Women: European Multicentre Case-Control Study," *BMJ* 321, no. 7254 (2000): 142–47.
2. J. L. Jones et al., "Risk Factors for Toxoplasma Gondii Infection in the United States," *Clinical Infectious Disease* 49, no. 6 (2009): 878–84.
3. J. Nohynek Gerhard et al., "Review: Toxicity and Human Health Risk of Hair Dyes," *Food and Chemical Toxicology* 42 (2004): 517–43.
4. Ibid.; Jennifer Connelly and Mark Malkin, "Environmental Risk Factors for Brain Tumors," *Current Neurology and Neuroscience Reports* 7, no. 3 (2007): 208–14.
5. L. Rylander et al., "Reproductive Outcomes Among Female Hairdressers," *Occupational and Environmental Medicine* 59 (2002): 517–22; Gerhard et al., "Review: Toxicity and Human Health Risk of Hair Dyes"; A. Chua-Gocheco, P. Bozzo, and A. Einarson, "Safety of Hair Products During Pregnancy," *Canadian Family Physician* 54 (2008): 1386–88.
6. Gerhard et al., "Review: Toxicity and Human Health Risk of Hair Dyes"; Chua-Gocheco, Bozzo, and Einarson, "Safety of Hair Products During Pregnancy."
7. H. Duong et al., "Maternal Use of Hot Tub and Major Structural Birth Defects," *Birth Defects Research Part A: Clinical and Molecular Teratology* 91 (2011): 836–41.
8. L. Suarez, M. Felkner, and K. Hendricks, "The Effect of Fever, Febrile Illnesses, and Heat Exposures on the Risk of Neural Tube Defects in a Texas-Mexico Border Population," *Birth Defects Research Part A: Clinical and Molecular Teratology* 70, no. 10 (2004): 815–19.
9. P. Dadvand et al., "Climate Extremes and the Length of Gestation," *Environmental Health Perspective* 119 (2011): 1449–53.
10. R. J. Barish, "In-Flight Radiation Exposure During Pregnancy," *Obstetrics & Gynecology* 103, no. 6 (2004): 1326–30.
11. Ibid.
12. M. Freeman et al, "Does Air Travel Affect Pregnancy Outcome?," *Archives of Gynecology and Obstetrics* 269, no. 4 (May, 2004): 274–77.

Chapter 10: Eating for Two? You Wish

1. T. O. School et al., "Gestational Weight Gain, Pregnancy Outcome, and Postpartum Weight Retention," *Obstetrics & Gynecology* 86 (1995): 423–27.

2. I. Thorsdottir and B. E. Birgisdottir, "Different Weight Gain in Women of Normal Weight Before Pregnancy: Postpartum Weight and Birth Weight," *Obstetrics and Gynecology* 92, no. 3 (1998): 377–83.

3. C. Ogden and M. Carroll, "Prevalence of Obesity Among Children and Adolescents: United States, Trends 1963–1965 through 2007–2008," *CDC Report* (June 2010).

4. L. Schack-Nielsen et al., "Gestational Weight Gain in Relation to Offspring Body Mass Index and Obesity from Infancy Through Adulthood," *International Journal of Obesity (2005)* 34, no. 1 (2010): 67–74.

5. A. A. Mamun et al., "Associations of Gestational Weight Gain with Offspring Body Mass Index and Blood Pressure at 21 Years of Age: Evidence from a Birth Cohort Study," *Circulation* 119, no. 13 (2009): 1720–27.

6. C. M. Olson, M. S. Strawderman, and B. A. Dennison, "Maternal Weight Gain During Pregnancy and Child Weight at Age 3 Years," *Maternal & Child Health Journal* 13, no. 6 (2009): 839–46.

7. B. H. Wrotniak et al., "Gestational Weight Gain and Risk of Overweight in the Offspring at Age 7 Y in a Multicenter, Multiethnic Cohort Study," *American Journal of Clinical Nutrition* 87, no. 6 (2008): 1818–24.

8. Sohyun Park et al., "Assessment of the Institute of Medicine Recommendations for Weight Gain During Pregnancy: Florida, 2004–2007," *Maternal & Child Health Journal* 15, no. 3 (2011): 289–301.

9. A. Tenovuo, "Neonatal Complications in Small-for-Gestational Age Neonates," *Journal of Perinatal Medicine* 16, no. 3 (1988): 197–203.

10. V. Giapros et al., "Morbidity and Mortality Patterns in Small-for-Gestational Age Infants Born Preterm," *Journal of Maternal-Fetal & Neonatal Medicine* 25, no. 2 (2012): 153–57.

11. P. Saenger et al., "Small for Gestational Age: Short Stature and Beyond," *Endocrine Reviews* 28, no. 2 (2007): 219–51.

12. S. Ng et al., "Risk Factors and Obstetric Complications of Large for Gestational Age Births with Adjustments for Community Effects: Results from a New Cohort Study," *BMC Public Health* 10 (2010): 460. http://www.ncbi.nlm.nih.gov/pmc/articles/PMC2921393/pdf/1471-2458-10-460.pdf

13. D. A. Savitz et al., "Gestational Weight Gain and Birth Outcome in Relation to Prepregnancy Body Mass Index and Ethnicity," *Annals of Epidemiology* 21 (2011): 78–85.

14. Ibid.

15. L. M. Bodnar et al., "Severe Obesity, Gestational Weight Gain, and Adverse Birth Outcomes," *American Journal of Clinical Nutrition* 91, no. 6 (2010): 1642–48.

16. Schack-Nielsen et al., "Gestational Weight Gain in Relation to Offspring Body Mass Index and Obesity from Infancy Through Adulthood."

Chapter 11: Pink and Blue

1. D. S. McKenna et al., "Gender-Related Differences in Fetal Heart Rate During First Trimester," *Fetal Diagnosis and Therapy* 21 (2006): 144–47.
2. P. Scheffer et al., "Reliability of Fetal Sex Determination Using Maternal Plasma," *Obstetrics & Gynecology* 115, no. 1 (2010): 117–26.
3. T. Shipp et al., "What Factors Are Associated with Parents' Desire to Know the Sex of Their Unborn Child?" *Birth* 31, no. 4 (2004): 272–79.
4. A. J. Wilcox, C. R. Weinberg, and D. D. Baird, "Timing of Sexual Intercourse in Relation to Ovulation—Effects on the Probability of Conception, Survival of the Pregnancy, and Sex of the Baby," *New England Journal of Medicine* 333, no. 23 (1995): 1517–21.

Chapter 12: Working Out and Resting Up

1. I. Streuling et al., "Physical Activity and Gestational Weight Gain: A Meta-Analysis of Intervention Trials," *BJOG* 118, no. 3 (2011): 278–84.
2. M. S. Kramer and S. W. McDonald, "Aerobic Exercise for Women During Pregnancy," *Cochrane Database of Systematic Reviews* 3 (2006).
3. C. M. Chiarello et al., "The Effects of an Exercise Program on Diastasis Recti Abdominis in Pregnant Women," *Journal of Women's Health Physical Therapy* 29, no. 1 (2005): 11–16.
4. K. Å. Salvesen, E. Hem, and J. Sundgot-Borgen, "Fetal Wellbeing May Be Compromised During Strenuous Exercise Among Pregnant Elite Athletes," *British Journal of Sports Medicine* 46 (2012): 279–83.
5. C. Meston et al., "Disorder of Orgasm in Women," *Journal of Sexual Medicine* 1, no. 1 (2004): 66–68.
6. P. C. Ko et al., "A Randomized Controlled Trial of Antenatal Pelvic Floor Exercises to Prevent and Treat Urinary Incontinence," *International Urogynecology Journal* 22, no. 1 (2011): 17–22.
7. J. Hay-Smith et al., "Pelvic Floor Muscle Training for Prevention and Treatment of Urinary and Faecal Incontinence in Antenatal and Postnatal Women," *Cochrane Database of Systematic Reviews* 4, article no. CD007471 (2008).
8. K. A. Salvesen and S. Mørkved, "Randomised Controlled Trial of Pelvic Floor Muscle Training During Pregnancy," *BMJ* 329, no. 7462 (2004): 378–80.
9. Y. C. et al., "Effects of a Prenatal Yoga Programme on the Discomforts of Pregnancy and Maternal Childbirth Self-Efficacy in Taiwan," *Midwifery* 26 (2010): e31–e36.
10. S. Chuntharapat, W. Petpichetchian, and U. Hatthakit, "Yoga During Pregnancy: Effects on Maternal Comfort, Labor Pain and Birth Outcomes," *Complementary Therapies in Clinical Practice* 14 (2008): 105–15.
11. B. N. Wikner and B. Källén, "Are Hypnotic Benzodiazepine Receptor Agonists Teratogenic in Humans?," *Journal of Clinical Psychopharmacology* 31, no. 3 (2011): 356–59.

12. L. H. Wang et al., "Increased Risk of Adverse Pregnancy Outcomes in Women Receiving Zolpidem During Pregnancy," *Clinical Pharmacology and Therapeutics* 88, no. 3 (2010): 369–74.

13. C. Ellington et al., "The Effect of Lateral Tilt on Maternal and Fetal Hemodynamic Variables," *Obstetrics & Gynecology* 77, no. 2 (1991): 201–3.

14. D. Farine and P. G. Seaward, "When It Comes to Pregnant Women Sleeping, Is Left Right?," *JOGC* 29, no. 10 (2007): 841–42.

15. T. Stacey et al., "Association Between Maternal Sleep Practices and Risk of Late Stillbirth: A Case-Control Study," *BMJ* 342 (2011): d3403. http://www.ncbi.nlm.nih.gov/pmc/articles/PMC3114953/pdf/bmj.d3403.pdf

Chapter 13: Drug Safety

1. C. Gedeon and G. Koren, "Designing Pregnancy Centered Medications: Drugs Which Do Not Cross the Human Placenta," *Placenta* 27, no. 8 (2006): 861–68.

2. L. M. De-Regil et al., "Effects and Safety of Periconceptional Folate Supplementation for Preventing Birth Defects" (Review), *Cochrane Database of Systematic Reviews* 10, article no. CD007950 (2010).

3. L. M. De-Regil, et al., "Effects and Safety of Periconceptional Folate Supplementation for Preventing Birth Defects (Review)." *Cochrane Database of Systematic Reviews* 2010, no. 10. Art. No.: CD007950.

4. A. R. Scialli et al., "A Review of the Literature on the Effects of Acetaminophen on Pregnancy Outcome," *Reproductive Toxicology* 30, no. 4 (2010): 495–507.

5. C. Rebordosa et al., "Acetaminophen Use During Pregnancy: Effects on Risk for Congenital Abnormalities," *American Journal of Obstetrics and Gynecology* 198 (2008): e1–e7.

6. B. Schick et al., "Abstract of the Ninth International Conference of the Organization of Teratology Information Services May 2–4, 1996 Salt Lake City, Utah, USA: Preliminary Analysis of First Trimester Exposure to Oxycodone and Hydrocodone," *Reproductive Toxicology* 10 (1996): 162.

7. C. S. Broussard et al., "Maternal Treatment with Opiod Analgesics and Risk for Birth Defects," *American Journal of Obstetrics and Gynecology* 204, no. 4 (2011): e1–e11.

8. A. H. Kline, R. J. Blattner, and M. Lunin, "Transplacental Effect of Tetracyclines on Teeth," *JAMA* 188 (1964): 178–80; J. R. Niebyl, "Antibiotics and Other Anti-infective Agents in Pregnancy and Lactation," *American Journal of Perinatology* 20, no. 8 (2003): 405–14.

9. E. J. Lammer et al., "Retinoic Acid Embryopathy," *New England Journal of Medicine* 313, no. 14 (1985): 837–41.

10. Steven Gabbe, Jennifer Niebyl, and Joe Leigh Simpson, *Obstetrics: Normal and Problem Pregnancies* (Philadelphia, PA: Churchill Livingstone, 2007).

Chapter 14: Premature Birth (and the Dangers of Bed Rest)

1. Author's calculations are based on the 2005 U.S. Natality Detail Files.

2. E. S. Potharst et al., "High Incidence of Multi-domain Disabilities in Very Preterm Children at Five Years of Age," *Journal of Pediatrics* 159, no. 1 (2011): 79–85.

3. For example: A. L. van Baar et al., "Functioning at School Age of Moderately Preterm Children Born at 32 to 36 Weeks' Gestational Age," *Pediatrics* 124, no. 1 (July 2009): 251–57; N. M. Talge et al., "Late-Preterm Birth and Its Association with Cognitive and Socioemotional Outcomes at 6 Years of Age," *Pediatrics* 126, no. 6 (2010): 1124–31.

4. Richard E. Behrman and Adrienne Stith Butler, eds., *Preterm Birth: Causes, Consequences, and Prevention* (Washington, D.C.: National Academies Press, 2007).

5. Steven Gabbe, Jennifer Niebyl, and Joe Leigh Simpson, *Obstetrics: Normal and Problem Pregnancies* (Philadelphia, PA: Churchill Livingstone, 2007).

6. D. Roberts and S. Dalziel, "Antenatal Corticosteroids for Accelerating Fetal Lung Maturation for Women at Risk of Preterm Birth," *Cochrane Database of Systematic Reviews* 3, article no. CD004454 (2006).

7. C. Sosa et al., "Bed Rest in Singleton Pregnancies for Preventing Preterm Birth," *Cochrane Database of Systematic Reviews* 1, article no. CD003581 (2004).

8. C. A. Crowther and S. Han, "Hospitalisation and Bed Rest for Multiple Pregnancy," *Cochrane Database of Systematic Reviews* 7, article no. CD000110 (2010).

9. C. Bigelow and J. Stone, "Bed Rest in Pregnancy," *Mount Sinai Journal of Medicine* 78, no. 2 (2011): 291–302.

10. J. Maloni, "Lack of Evidence for Prescription of Antepartum Bed Rest," *Expert Review in Obstetrics and Gynecology* 6, no. 4 (2011): 385–93.

11. Bigelow and Stone, "Bed Rest in Pregnancy."

12. N. S. Fox et al., "Research: The Recommendation for Bed Rest in the Setting of Arrested Preterm Labor and Premature Rupture of Membranes," *American Journal of Obstetrics and Gynecology* 200 (2009): 165.e1, 165.e6.

Chapter 15: High-Risk Pregnancy

1. Many of the details about conditions in this chapter come from Steven Gabbe, Jennifer Niebyl, and Joe Leigh Simpson, *Obstetrics: Normal and Problem Pregnancies* (Philadelphia, PA: Churchill Livingstone, 2007). Other references are included where appropriate.

2. D. A. Wing, R. H. Paul, and L. K. Millar, "Management of the Symptomatic Placenta Previa: A Randomized, Controlled Trial of Inpatient Versus Outpatient Expectant Management," *American Journal of Obstetrics and Gynecology* 175, no. 4 (1996): 806–11; J. R. Mouer, "Placenta Previa: Antepartum Conservative Management, Inpatient Versus Outpatient," *American Journal of Obstetrics and Gynecology* 170, no. 6 (1994): 1683–85; S. Droste and K. Keil, "Expectant Management of Placenta Previa: Cost-Benefit Analysis of Outpatient Treatment," *American Journal of Obstetrics and Gynecology* 170, no. 5 (1994): 1254–57.

3. E. Sakornbut, L. Leeman, and P. Fontaine, "Late Pregnancy Bleeding," *American Family Physician* 75, no. 8 (2007): 1199.
4. Gabbe, Niebyl, and Simpson, *Obstetrics: Normal and Problem Pregnancies*; N. Alwan, D. J. Tuffnell, and J. West, "Treatments for Gestational Diabetes," *Cochrane Database of Systematic Reviews* 3, article no. CD003395 (2009).
5. Alwan, Tuffnell, and West, "Treatments for Gestational Diabetes."
6. Gabbe, Niebyl, and Simpson, *Obstetrics: Normal and Problem Pregnancies*; J. Iams et al., "The Length of the Cervix and the Risk of Spontaneous Premature Delivery," *New England Journal of Medicine* 334 (1996): 567–72.
7. A. J. Drakeley, D. Roberts, and Z. Alfirevic, "Cervical Stitch (Cerclage) for Preventing Pregnancy Loss in Women," *Cochrane Database of Systematic Reviews* 1 (2003).
8. Ibid.
9. S. M. Althuisius et al., "Cervical Incompetence Prevention Randomized Cerclage Trial: Emergency Cerclage with Bed Rest Versus Bed Rest Alone," *American Journal of Obstetrics & Gynecology* 189, no. 4 (2003): 907–10; S. M. Althuisius et al., "Final Results of the Cervical Incompetence Prevention Randomized Cerclage Trial (CIPRACT): Therapeutic Cerclage with Bed Rest Versus Bed Rest Alone," *American Journal of Obstetrics and Gynecology* 185, no. 5 (2001): 1106–12.
10. Gabbe, Niebyl, and Simpson, *Obstetrics: Normal and Problem Pregnancies*.
11. Ibid.
12. L. Duley et al., "Antiplatelet Agents for Preventing Pre-eclampsia and Its Complications," *Cochrane Database of Systematic Reviews* 2 (2007).
13. G. J. Hofmeyr et al., "Calcium Supplementation During Pregnancy for Preventing Hypertensive Disorders and Related Problems," *Cochrane Database of Systematic Reviews* 8 (2010).

Chapter 16: I'm Going to Be Pregnant Forever, Right?

1. R. Mittendorf et al., "The Length of Uncomplicated Human Gestation," *Obstetrics & Gynecology* 75, no. 6 (1990): 929–32.
2. This graph was constructed by the authors based on the 2008 U.S. Natality Detail Files.
3. P. Rozenberg, F. Goffinet, and M. Hessabi, "Comparison of the Bishop Score, Ultrasonographically Measured Cervical Length, and Fetal Fibronectin Assay in Predicting Time Until Delivery and Type of Delivery at Term," *American Journal of Obstetrics and Gynecology* 182 (2000): 108–13; G. Ramanathan et al., "Ultrasound Examination at 37 Weeks' Gestation in the Prediction of Pregnancy Outcome: The Value of Cervical Assessment," *Ultrasound in Obstetrics & Gynecology* 22, no. 6 (2003): 598–603. A more accurate way to say this is to note that in Rozenberg et al., cervical length and the overall Bishop Score (including everything) had the same predictive power.
4. Ramanathan et al., "Ultrasound Examination at 37 Weeks' Gestation in the Prediction of Pregnancy Outcome."

5. E. Strobel et al., "Bishop Score and Ultrasound Assessment of the Cervix for Prediction of Time to Onset of Labor and Time to Delivery in Prolonged Pregnancy," *Ultrasound in Obstetrics & Gynecology* 28, no. 3 (2006): 298–305.

6. J. D. Iams et al., "The Preterm Prediction Study: Can Low-Risk Women Destined for Spontaneous Preterm Birth Be Identified?," *American Journal of Obstetrics and Gynecology* 184, no. 4 (2001): 652–55.

7. Steven Gabbe, Jennifer Niebyl, and Joe Leigh Simpson, *Obstetrics: Normal and Problem Pregnancies* (Philadelphia, PA: Churchill Livingstone, 2007).

Chapter 17: Labor Induction

1. Steven Gabbe, Jennifer Niebyl, and Joe Leigh Simpson, *Obstetrics: Normal and Problem Pregnancies* (Philadelphia, PA: Churchill Livingstone, 2007).

2. Z. Alfirevic, A. J. Kelly, and T. Dowswell, "Intravenous Oxytocin Alone for Cervical Ripening and Induction of Labour," *Cochrane Database of Systematic Reviews* 4 (2009).

3. Ibid.; A. J. Kelly et al., "Vaginal Prostaglandin (PGE2 and PGF2a) for Induction of Labour at Term," *Cochrane Database of Systematic Reviews* 4 (2009).

4. A. M. Gülmezoglu, C. A. Crowther, and P. Middleton, "Induction of Labour for Improving Birth Outcomes for Women at or Beyond Term," *Cochrane Database of Systematic Reviews* 4 (2006); M. Thorsell et al., "Induction of Labor and the Risk for Emergency Cesarean Section in Nulliparous and Multiparous Women," *AOGS* 90, no. 10 (2011): 1094–99.

5. Gabbe, Niebyl, and Simpson. *Obstetrics: Normal and Problem Pregnancies.*

6. D. Elsandabesee, S. Majumdar, and S. Sinha, "Obstetricians' Attitudes Towards 'Isolated' Oligohydraminos at Term," *Journal of Obstetrics and Gynaecology* 27, no. 6 (2007): 574–76.

7. E. Mozurkewich et al., "Indications for Induction of Labour: A Best-Evidence Review," *BJOG* 116, no. 5 (2009): 626–36.

8. S. Ek et al., "Oligohydraminos in Uncomplicated Pregnancies Beyond 40 Completed Weeks," *Fetal Diagnosis and Therapy* 20 (2005): 182–85.

9. J. Zhang et al., "Isolated Oligohydraminos Is Not Associated with Adverse Perinatal Outcomes," *BJOG* 111, no. 3 (2004): 220–25.

10. N. Melamed et al., "Perinatal Outcome in Pregnancies Complicated by Isolated Oligohydraminos Diagnosed Before 37 Weeks of Gestation," *American Journal of Obstetrics and Gynecology* 205 (2011): 241.e1–e6.

11. A. F. Nabhan and Y. A. Abdelmoula, "Review Article: Amniotic Fluid Index Versus Single Deepest Vertical Pocket: A Meta-Analysis of Randomized Controlled Trials," *International Journal of Gynecology and Obstetrics* 104 (2009): 184–88.

12. G. J. Hofmeyr and A. M. Gülmezoglu, "Maternal Hydration for Increasing Amniotic Fluid Volume in Oligohydraminos and Normal Amniotic Fluid Volume," *Cochrane Database of Systematic Reviews* 1 (2002).

13. Q. Xi et al., "Clinical Study on Detecting False Non-Reactive of Non-Stress Test by Improved Acoustic Stimulation," *Archives of Gynecology and Obstetrics* 284, no. 2 (2011): 271–74.

14. K. E. McCarthy and D. Narrigan, "Is There Scientific Support for the Use of Juice to Facilitate the Nonstress Test?," *Journal of Obstetric, Gynecologic, & Neonatal Nursing* 24, no. 4 (1995): 303–7.

15. H. G. Hall, L. G. McKenna, and D. L. Griffiths, "Discussion: Complementary and Alternative Medicine for Induction of Labour," *Women and Birth* 25, no. 3 (September 2012): 142–48.

16. M. Simpson et al., "Raspberry Leaf in Pregnancy: Its Safety and Efficacy in Labor," *Journal of Midwifery & Women's Health* 46, no. 2 (2001): 51–59.

17. D. Dove and P. Johnson, "Oral Evening Primrose Oil: Its Effect on Length of Pregnancy and Selected Intrapartum Outcomes in Low-Risk Nulliparous Women," *Journal of Nurse-Midwifery* 44, no. 3 (1999): 320–24.

18. P. C. Tan et al., "Effect of Coitus at Term on Length of Gestation, Induction of Labor, and Mode of Delivery," *Obstetrics & Gynecology* 108, no. 1 (2006): 134–40.

19. P. C. Tan, C. M. Yow, and S. Z. Omar, "Effect of Coital Activity on Onset of Labor in Women Scheduled for Labor Induction," *Obstetrics & Gynecology* 110, no. 4 (2007): 820–26.

20. C. A. Smith and C. A. Crowther, "Acupuncture for Induction of Labour," *Cochrane Database of Systematic Reviews* 1 (2004).

21. J. Modlock, B. B. Nielsen, and N. Uldbjerg, "Acupuncture for the Induction of Labour: A Double-Blind Randomised Controlled Study," *BJOG* 117, no. 10 (2010): 1255–61.

22. C. A. Smith, C. A. Crowther, C. T. Collins, and M. E. Coyle, "Acupuncture to Induce Labor: A Randomized Controlled Trial," *Obstetrics and Gynecology* 112, no. 5 (2008): 1067–74.

23. J. Kavanagh, A. J. Kelly, and J. Thomas, "Breast Stimulation for Cervical Ripening and Induction of Labour," *Cochrane Database of Systematic Reviews* 3, article no. CD003392 (2005).

24. M. Boulvain, C. M. Stan, and O. Irion, "Membrane Sweeping for Induction of Labour," *Cochrane Database of Systematic Reviews* 1 (2005).

Chapter 18: The Labor Numbers

1. E. A. Friedman, "Primigravid Labor; a Graphicostatistical Analysis," *Obstetrics & Gynecology* 6, no. 6 (1955): 567–89.

2. J. Zhang, J. F. Troendle, and M. K. Yancey, "Reassessing the Labor Curve in Nulliparous Women," *American Journal of Obstetrics and Gynecology* 187, no. 4 (2002): 824–28.

3. Steven Gabbe, Jennifer Niebyl, and Joe Leigh Simpson, *Obstetrics: Normal and Problem Pregnancies* (Philadelphia, PA: Churchill Livingstone, 2007).

4. M. Westgren et al., "Spontaneous Cephalic Version of Breech Presentation in the Last Trimester," *BJOG* 92 (1985): 19–22.

5. G. J. Hofmeyr and K. Regina, "External Cephalic Version for Breech Presentation at Term," *Cochrane Database of Systematic Reviews* 1, article no. CD000083 (1996).
6. J. M. Dodd et al., "Planned Elective Repeat Caesarean Section Versus Planned Vaginal Birth for Women with a Previous Caesarean Birth," *Cochrane Database of Systematic Reviews* 4, article no. CD 004224 (2004).
7. Caroline Crowther et al., "Planned Vaginal Birth or Elective Repeat Caesarean: Patient Preference Restricted Cohort with Nested Randomised Trial," *PLOS Medicine* 9, no. 3 (2012): e1001192.
8. E. Mozurkewich and E. Hutton, "Elective Repeat Caesarean Delivery Versus Trial of Labor: A Meta-Analysis of the Literature from 1989 to 1999," *American Journal of Obstetrics and Gynecology* 183 (2000): 1187–97.

Chapter 19: To Epidural or Not to Epidural?

1. M. Anim-Somuah, R. M. Smyth, and L. Jones, "Epidural Versus Non-Epidural or No Analgesia in Labour," *Cochrane Database of Systematic Reviews* 12 (2011).
2. Both this information and the data for moms come from the above review.
3. S. K. Sharma, "Epidural Analgesia During Labor and Maternal Fever," *Current Opinion in Anaesthesiology* 13, no. 3 (2000): 257–60.
4. M. Van de Velde et al., "Original Article: Ten Years of Experience with Accidental Dural Puncture and Post-Dural Puncture Headache in a Tertiary Obstetric Anaesthesia Department," *International Journal of Obstetric Anesthesia* 17 (2008): 329–35.
5. C. A. Smith, C. T. Collins, and C. A. Crowther, "Aromatherapy for Pain Management in Labour," *Cochrane Database of Systematic Reviews* 7 (2011).
6. C. A. Smith et al., "Acupuncture or Acupressure for Pain Management in Labour," *Cochrane Database of Systematic Reviews* 7 (2011)
7. S. H. Cho, H. Lee, and E. Ernst, "Acupuncture for Pain Relief in Labour: A Systematic Review and Meta-Analysis," *BJOG* 117, no. 8 (2010): 907–20.

Chapter 20: Beyond Pain Relief

1. S. L. Buchanan et al., "Planned Early Birth Versus Expectant Management for Women with Preterm Prelabour Rupture of Membranes Prior to 37 Weeks' Gestation for Improving Pregnancy Outcome," *Cochrane Database of Systematic Reviews* 3 (2010); M. E. Hannah et al., "Induction of Labor Compared with Expectant Management for Prelabor Rupture of the Membranes at Term," TermPROM Study Group, *New England Journal of Medicine* 334, no. 16 (1996): 1005–10.
2. C. Mendelson, "The Aspiration of Stomach Contents into the Lungs During Obstetric Anesthesia," *American Journal of Obstetrics and Gynecology* 52 (1946): 191–205.
3. J. Hawkins et al., "Anesthesia-Related Maternal Mortality in the United States: 1979–2002," *Obstetrics & Gynecology* 117, no. 1 (2011): 69–74.

4. D. Maharaj, "Review: Eating and Drinking in Labor: Should It Be Allowed?,"*European Journal of Obstetrics and Gynecology* 146 (2009): 3–7.

5. M. Kubli et al., "An Evaluation of Isotonic 'Sport Drinks' During Labor," *Anesthesia and Analgesia* 94, no. 2 (2002): 404.

6. Ibid.

7. S. K. McGrath and J. H. Kennell, "A Randomized Controlled Trial of Continuous Labor Support for Middle-Class Couples: Effect on Cesarean Delivery Rates," *Birth: Issues in Perinatal Care* 35, no. 2 (2008): 92–97.

8. J. Kennell et al., "Continuous Emotional Support During Labor in a U.S. Hospital: A Randomized Controlled Trial," *JAMA* 265, no. 17 (1991): 2197–2201.

9. Z. Alfirevic, D. Devane, and G. M. Gyte, "Continuous Cardiotocography (CTG) as a Form of Electronic Fetal Monitoring (EFM) for Fetal Assessment During Labour," *Cochrane Database of Systematic Reviews* 3 (2006).

10. Z. Nachum et al., "Comparison Between Amniotomy, Oxytocin or Both for Augmentation of Labor in Prolonged Latent Phase: A Randomized Controlled Trial," *Reproductive Biology & Endocrinology* 8 (2010): 136–43; S. Wei et al., "Early Amniotomy and Early Oxytocin for Prevention of, or Therapy for, Delay in First Stage Spontaneous Labour Compared with Routine Care," *Cochrane Database of Systematic Reviews* 2 (2009).

11. G. Carroli and L. Mignini, "Episiotomy for Vaginal Birth," *Cochrane Database of Systematic Reviews* 1 (2009).

12. Author's calculations are from the U.S. Natality Detail Files.

13. A. Cotter, A. Ness, and J. Tolosa, "Prophylactic Oxytocin for the Third Stage of Labor," *Cochrane Database of Systematic Reviews* 4 (2001); C. M. Begley et al., "Active Versus Expectant Management for Women in the Third Stage of Labor," *Cochrane Database of Systematic Reviews* 11 (2011).

14. Begley et al., "Active Versus Expectant Management for Women in the Third Stage of Labor."

Chapter 21: The Aftermath

1. H. Rabe, G. Reynolds, and J. Diaz-Rossello, "Early Versus Delayed Umbilical Cord Clamping in Preterm Infants," *Cochrane Database of Systematic Reviews* 4, article no. CD003248 (2004).

2. S. J. McDonald and P. Middleton, "Effect of Timing of Umbilical Cord Clamping of Term Infants on Maternal and Neonatal Outcomes," *Cochrane Database of Systematic Reviews* 2 (2008).

3. American Academy of Pediatrics Committee on Fetus and Newborn, "Controversies Concerning Vitamin K and the Newborn," *Pediatrics* 112, no. 1 (2003): 191–92; J. A. Ross and S. M. Davies, "Vitamin K Prophylaxis and Childhood Cancer," *Medical and Pediatric Oncology* 34, no. 6 (2000): 434–37.

4. J. Golding, M. Paterson, and L. J. Kinlen, "Factors Associated with Childhood Cancer in a National Cohort Study," *British Journal of Cancer* 62, no. 2 (1990): 304–8.

5. J. Golding et al., "Childhood Cancer, Intramuscular Vitamin K, and Pethidine Given During Labour," *BMJ* 305, no. 6849 (1992): 341–46.

6. G. J. Draper et al., "Intramuscular Vitamin K and Childhood Cancer [with Reply]," *BMJ* 305, no. 6855 (1992): 709–11.

7. H. Ekelund et al., "Administration of Vitamin K to Newborn Infants and Childhood Cancer," *BMJ* 307, no. 6896 (1993): 89–91; J. A. Ross and S. M. Davies, "Vitamin K Prophylaxis and Childhood Cancer," *Medical and Pediatric Oncology* 34, no. 6 (2000): 434–37.

8. *American Academy of Pediatrics Committee on Fetus and Newborn, "Controversies Concerning Vitamin K and the Newborn."*

9. E. K. Darling and H. McDonald, "A Meta-Analysis of the Efficacy of Ocular Prophylactic Agents Used for the Prevention of Gonococcal and Chlamydial Ophthalmia Neonatorum," *Journal of Midwifery & Women's Health* 55, no. 4 (2010): 319–27.

10. B. A. Armson, "Umbilical Cord Blood Banking: Implications for Perinatal Care Providers," *JOGC* 27, no. 3 (2005): 263–90; G. J. Annas, "Waste and Longing—The Legal Status of Placental-Blood Banking," *New England Journal of Medicine* 340, no. 19 (1999): 1521–24.

11. A. J. French et al., "Development of Human Cloned Blastocysts Following Somatic Cell Nuclear Transfer with Adult Fibroblasts," *Stem Cells* 26, no. 2 (2008): 485–93.

Chapter 22: Home Birth: Progressive or Regressive? And Who Cleans the Tub?

1. Author's calculations are based on the 2008 U.S. Natality Detail Files.

2. J. R. Wax et al., "Maternal and Newborn Outcomes in Planned Home Birth Vs Planned Hospital Births: A Metaanalysis," *American Journal of Obstetrics and Gynecology* 203, no. 3 (2010): 243.e1, 243.e8.

3. Birthplace in England Collaborative Group, "Perinatal and Maternal Outcomes by Planned Place of Birth for Healthy Women with Low Risk Pregnancies: The Birthplace in England National Prospective Cohort Study," *BMJ* 343 (2011): d7400.

4. Wax et al., "Maternal and Newborn Outcomes in Planned Home Birth Vs Planned Hospital Births."

5. A. de Jonge et al., "Perinatal Mortality and Morbidity in a Nationwide Cohort of 529,688 Low-Risk Planned Home and Hospital Births," *BJOG* 116, no. 9 (2009): 1177–84; A. C. Evers et al., "Perinatal Mortality and Severe Morbidity in Low and High Risk Term Pregnancies in the Netherlands: Prospective Cohort Study," *BMJ* 341 (2010): c5639.

6. J. W. Y. Pang et al., "Outcomes of Planned Home Births in Washington State: 1989–1996," *Obstetrics & Gynecology* 100, no. 2 (2002): 253–59; P. A. Janssen et al., "Outcomes of Planned Home Birth with Registered

Midwife Versus Planned Hospital Birth with Midwife or Physician," *CMAJ* 181, no. 6 (2009): 377–83.
7. Birthplace in England Collaborative Group, "Perinatal and Maternal Outcomes by Planned Place of Birth for Healthy Women with Low Risk Pregnancies."

Appendix

1. S. M. Gilboa et al., "Use of Antihistamine Medications During Early Pregnancy and Isolated Major Malformations," *Birth Defects Research Part A* 85, no. 2 (2009): 137–50.
2. O. Diav-Citrin et al., "Pregnancy Outcome After Gestational Exposure to Loratadine or Antihistamines: A Prospective Controlled Cohort Study," *Journal of Allergy and Clinical Immunology* 111, no. 6 (2003): 1239–43.
3. M. Sarkar et al., "Pregnancy Outcome Following Gestational Exposure to Azithromycin," *BMC Pregnancy and Childbirth* 6 (2006): 18; B. Bar-Oz et al., "Pregnancy Outcome After Gestational Exposure to the New Macrolides: A Prospective Multi-Center Observational Study," *European Journal of Obstetrics, Gynecology, and Reproductive Biology* 141, no. 1 (2008): 31–34.
4. G. G. Nahum, K. Uhl, and D. L. Kennedy, "Antibiotic Use in Pregnancy and Lactation: What Is and Is Not Known About Teratogenic and Toxic Risks," *Obstetrics & Gynecology* 107, no. 5 (2006): 1120–38.
5. S. Gentile, "Drug Treatment for Mood Disorders in Pregnancy," *Current Opinion in Psychiatry* 24, no. 1 (2011): 34–40.
6. O. Diav-Citrin et al., "The Safety of Proton Pump Inhibitors in Pregnancy: A Multicentre Prospective Controlled Study," *Alimentary Pharmacology & Therapeutics* 21, no. 3 (2005): 269–75; A. Ruigómez et al., "Use of Cimetidine, Omeprazole, and Ranitidine in Pregnant Women and Pregnancy Outcomes," *American Journal of Epidemiology* 150, no. 5 (1999): 476–81; S. K. Gill et al., "The Safety of Proton Pump Inhibitors (PPIs) in Pregnancy: A Meta-Analysis," *American Journal of Gastroenterology* 104, no. 6 (2009): 1541–45.
7. H. Garbis et al., "Pregnancy Outcome After Exposure to Ranitidine and Other H-2 Blockers," *Reproductive Toxocology* 19, no. 4 (2005): 453–58.
8. M. Thomas and S. M. Wiesman, "Calcium Supplementation During Pregnancy and Lactation: Effects on the Mother and the Fetus," *American Journal of Obstetrics and Gynecology* 194, no. 4 (2006): 937–45.
9. W. O. Cooper et al., "Major Congenital Malformations After First-Trimester Exposure to ACE Inhibitors, *New England Journal of Medicine* 354, no. 23 (2006): 2443–51; G. Briggs and B. Pharm, "Drug Effects on the Fetus and Breast-Fed Infant," *Clinical Obstetrics & Gynecology* 45, no. 1 (2002): 6–21.
10. L. A. Magee et al., "The Safety of Calcium Channel Blockers in Human Pregnancy: A Prospective, Multicenter Cohort Study," *American Journal of Obstetrics and Gynecology* 174, no. 3 (1996): 823–28; C. Weber-Schoendorfer et al., "The Safety of Calcium Channel Blockers During

Pregnancy: A Prospective, Multicenter, Observational Study," *Reproductive Toxicology* 26, no. 1 (2008): 24–30.

11. P. S. Pollack et al., "Pregnancy Outcomes After Maternal Exposure to Simvastatin and Lovastatin," *Birth Defects Research Part A: Clinical and Molecular Teratology* 73, no. 11 (2005): 888–96; N. Taguchi et al., "Prenatal Exposure to HMG-Coa Reductase Inhibitors: Effects on Fetal and Neonatal Outcomes," *Reproductive Toxicology* 26, no. 2 (2008): 175–77.

12. R. K. Hernandez et al., "Nonsteroidal Anti-inflammatory Drug Use Among Women and the Risk of Birth Defects," *American Journal of Obstetrics and Gynecology* 206, no. 3 (2012): 1–8.

13. R. Padmanabhan and D. J. Pallot, "Aspirin-Alcohol Interaction in the Production of Cleft Palate and Limb Malformations in the TO Mouse," *Teratology* 51, no. 6 (1995): 404–17; R. T. Robertson, H. L. Allen, and D. L. Bokelman, "Aspirin: Teratogenic Evaluation in the Dog," *Teratology* 20, no. 2 (1979): 313–20.

14. G. Turner and E. Collins, "Fetal Effects of Regular Salicylate Ingestion in Pregnancy," *Lancet* 2, no. 7930 (1975): 338–39.

15. D. Slone et al., "Aspirin and Congenital Malformations," *Lancet* 1, no. 7974 (1976): 1373–75.

Index